THE <u>REAL</u>
FORBIDDEN FRUIT

"Jeff Popick is a passionate man with a compelling message. In The Real Forbidden Fruit he describes, often with great brilliance, the reasons he and many others feel both a moral and intellectual imperative to be vegan.

As outspoken as he is thoughtful, Jeff Popick isn't about to sit back in resignation and watch humanity descend ever deeper into darkness.

Shining like a torch, his writings come from deeply held convictions and profound concern for the welfare of all sentient beings."

~ John Robbins, author of
Diet For A New America
and *Healthy At 100*

THE *REAL* FORBIDDEN FRUIT

How Meat Destroys Paradise
And How Veganism
Can Get It Back

Jeff Popick

The Real Forbidden Fruit:
How Meat Destroys Paradise And How Veganism Can Get It Back
Jeff Popick

Published by: VeganWorld Publishing
1083 N. Collier Blvd.
Box 404
Marco Island, FL 34145
E-Mail: publisher@veganworld.com

Library of Congress Control Number: 2007921577

ISBN: 978-0-9671518-0-9 Hardcover
ISBN: 978-0-9671518-1-6 Paperback
ISBN: 978-0-9671518-2-3 Audio Book
ISBN: 978-0-9671518-3-0 E-Book

Printed in the United States of America

0 9 8 7 6 5 4 3 2 1

This book has been printed on 60% recycled, acid-free paper using soy-based inks.

Table of Contents

Disclaimers Without Fine Print

I believe that veganism is the healthiest way of life and can prevent, cure and even reverse some of the many debilitating, degenerative and deadly conditions that are proliferating in our world today. My reasons are explained in detail in this book.

However, because our society, including the medical profession, is influenced in large part by the meat and dairy industries (for reasons that are also explained herein), I am compelled to warn you to seek the advice of a doctor before changing your diet, medication or exercise regimen. I strongly recommend you find a doctor who is either vegan or vegetarian, or at the very least, one who understands the health benefits of such a lifestyle.

I also encourage you to pursue truth and become an expert in the things that affect your life and health. You will be in a better position to make future decisions.

Foreword

Today, in my opinion, the Earth is poised on the brink of disaster. For many years I've been concerned at the rate we are trashing the planet. At the rate we are destroying rain forests, they will cease to exist in our lifetime.

The Earth's topsoil is being displaced by our farming practices. In three hundred years, the United States has lost the majority of topsoil that was here when the boat people arrived. Lost topsoil and chemical runoff draining down the Mississippi have caused an area in the Gulf of Mexico as large as the State of New Jersey to be devoid of life.

If these problems are not enough, we can add global warming. The millions of tons of carbon being exhausted into the atmosphere have changed the temperature on the planet. The Earth is warming to the point where the temperature of the water off the coast of California has increased four degrees in the last forty years. The ice fields are shrinking at a rate of about fourteen thousand square miles of ice pack each year. Studies indicate the Arctic ice fields have eroded about forty percent since the 1950s. Melting at today's rate would mean the Arctic ice cap would disappear within eighteen years.

The Antarctic ice cap is also deteriorating. Recently, a piece of the South Pole ice pack, which is one and a half times larger than the State of Rhode Island, broke off and is drifting north into warm water, where it will melt. There is concern that if a larger section breaks off and moves north, it could raise the levels of the world's oceans by seventeen feet.

You look at all of these things and you ask yourself, what in the world does this have to do with eating a vegan diet? The answer is: everything.

The population has exceeded six billion people and is doubling every fifty years. There is great concern about how we are going to feed a hungry world. Yet we continue to waste valuable food (grain) and energy to raise animals for food. The fact is, it takes at least twelve pounds of grain to produce one pound of meat.

Global warming, loss of valuable top soil, feeding a hungry world and not wasting energy are at the core of the reasons for adopting a plant-based diet. The largest area of change available to planners in the short term to avert mass starvation will be a change in the global diet.

It makes no difference if the reason you are exploring a plant-based diet is your love of animals, your concern for the environment or just your own health; this book has the answers. Jeff Popick has taken a very complex and personal issue and put it in a factual, easy-to-read form that can change your life. He has also given us the justification for our action as it affects all of creation.

The Real Forbidden Fruit has something for everyone. Jeff shows the interconnected nature of power, greed, violence, freedom, love and many other aspects of our lives as they relate to a vegan diet. I was totally drawn into the fabric of this book. When I finished reading it I knew what the reader should do to make a start on the path to a better life before it is too late for our children and grandchildren.

I wish I had read this book twenty years ago. Then I could have started on my own path toward better health for the planet, the animals and myself. I pray we change in time to save the future generations.

Howard Lyman

Howard Lyman is a fourth generation cattle rancher turned vegan who achieved notoriety when his explanation on *Oprah* about how beef is produced caused Ms. Winfrey to exclaim, "It has just stopped me cold from eating another burger!"

The resulting lawsuit brought by a group of Texas cattlemen was finally dismissed "with prejudice" (meaning it cannot be appealed or filed again anywhere, including the Supreme Court) in August 2002.

Lyman is former president of EarthSave International and the International Vegetarian Union, and is the best-selling author of *Mad Cowboy: Plain Truth from the Cattle Rancher Who Won't Eat Meat*.

As Founder/President of *Voice for a Viable Future*, Lyman spends his time writing and speaking on the calamitous ramifications of a meat-based economy, for which his background in agribusiness prepared him so well.

His latest book is *NO MORE BULL! The Mad Cowboy Targets America's Worst Enemy: Our Diet*.

Introduction

Grant me one small favor and I will, in return, grant you a tremendous favor. All you need to do is answer this one question: Would you rather live your life in a paradise or in a dystopia? I'm going to assume that you would choose paradise, since virtually every sane human on the planet would.

Most people, maybe even you, think veganism, the purest form of vegetarianism, is about healthy eating. But that would be like thinking skydiving is about transportation. Sure, skydiving will get you from Point A to Point B, but that's hardly the reason for willingly jumping out of working airplanes.

"Kindness," "compassion," "caring" and "empathy" are words that begin to approach the complete meaning and definition of veganism. Perhaps one word that can be used to sum this all up is "humanity," and a good example of humanity in action is the golden rule: Do unto all others as you would like all others to do unto you.

Most people subscribe to the principles of the golden rule, yet most of these same people kill and eat animals, clearly a violation of that rule. We say we love animals, yet we eat animals. Hmmm. With friends like that, animals don't need any enemies. Many of us even believe we live our lives peaceably and consider "might over right" to be barbaric, then go out to a restaurant and eat a defenseless animal. I understand why people eat meat; they have acquired a taste for it. But not everything that tastes or feels good is right. It would probably feel good to slap that coworker who stole your ideas and got promoted over you, but it wouldn't be right. (That might be a bad example, but you get the idea.) No matter how civilized we like to think we are, when we sit down to a breakfast of ham and eggs or a lunch of a chicken sandwich or a dinner of surf and turf, we – not them over there – *we* perpetuate the barbaric, violent, diseased world that we live in today. This applies to all, no matter how plain or fancy the restaurant or how expensive the real estate upon which the ovens sit. Humanity, peace and happiness are distorted through the lens of hypocrisy when veganism is abandoned.

From this it becomes clear that other seemingly easy words, such as "truth" and "love," will also need some functional clarification. This book will provide that.

Our educational systems teach nothing of humanity, and then we wonder why our society has become a violence factory. Our schools also teach nothing of empathy, and then we're surprised that nobody gives a damn about anything or anyone other than themselves.

From our Judeo-Christian society's standpoint, the Biblical definition for Heaven on Earth (or utopia or paradise, whichever you prefer) is: "The wolf and the lamb shall feed together, and the lion shall eat straw like the ox: and dust shall be the serpent's food. They shall not hurt nor destroy in all My holy mountain, saith the Lord" (Isaiah 65:25). Moreover, at the very beginning of Creation, God clearly tells mankind that he has given us plants for food. Yet today, mankind worships God but ignores one of His earliest, clearest and most direct mandates. To make matters worse, mankind then doesn't understand, or chooses to not understand, where all its problems are coming from.

So where did we go wrong and how do we get back? I'm glad you asked. The intention of this book is to introduce you to some of the concepts behind veganism, show you some of the many disastrous ramifications of not being vegan, as well as the enormous benefits in choosing to be vegan. While we all have many painful problems today, it is this author's ardent position that our world was actually created to be a paradise. The world's pain, and even *your* pain, stems from the embracement of meat and dairy. In no uncertain terms, meat is to hell as veganism is to heaven. This book will serve as a roadmap back to paradise, but be warned, you will have to walk each mile yourself, and some of it is uphill.

Veganism is really about love, truth, happiness, peace and harmony, and kinship amongst all the Earth's inhabitants. Further, a vegan way of life offers deep spirituality and a real connection to God. Oh, and by the way, veganism is also the healthiest way of eating and a virtual sure thing for weight control. However, good health is a spillover benefit and is merely one tiny feature in the grand landscape of veganism. Veganism is not so much a guide to health as it is a guide to life. Veganism is the asphalt on the road to paradise.

And, speaking of which, here is my favor to you: The road to paradise.

"To become vegetarian is to step into the stream which leads to Nirvana." – The Buddha

Part One

"Sit down before fact like a little child, and be prepared to give up every preconceived notion, follow humbly wherever and to whatever abyss nature leads, or you shall learn nothing."

– T. H. Huxley

Chapter 1

Solutions

I am going to go out on a limb and make the claim that just about every single person on the planet believes killing is wrong. For the very rare few who overtly disbelieve this, there are jails. "Thou shalt not kill" is an almost universally agreed-upon principle, yet almost everyone eats animals. This begs one question: Huh?

There is always a reason why problems occur. However, if we are unable or unwilling to see that reason, the first problem flourishes and often creates more problems in its wake. There is a technique, an art, if you will, to real problem solving. The problem is (no pun intended) that all people on the planet face problems, yet very few have spent any time learning how to solve problems. Trying to solve a problem without knowing how to solve problems is problematic; one problem causing more problems, which then cause more problems.

In mathematics, there is often only one right answer. For instance, 7 x 7 = 49. But there are an unlimited number of wrong answers (specifically 0 through 48, and 50 through infinity in this instance). Similar to math, life's problems can also be solved, but there are always more wrong answers than right answers. The odds of you arbitrarily picking the right answer are stacked astronomically against you. There may very well be a single answer, a simple truth actually, but unless we know how to find it, the chances of doing so are slim or none – and slim just left town.

Problems and their solutions have fascinated me from the time I was a small child. Since I was the baby in the family, and everyone was always telling me to shut up, I found myself doing a lot of listening. I would hear seemingly intelligent people discuss politics and wonder why they could disagree so ardently on various issues. "If both sides are intelligent," I wondered, "shouldn't they be coming up with the same answer, the correct answer?"

I realized that everyone has *an* answer, but most are formulated in the absence of the art of problem solving and are, therefore, wrong. So I began to wonder what the real answers were to some of the commonly discussed problems, such as gun control, abortion and deficit spending, and I discovered there are no real answers to these problems. These are nonissues generated by inept problem solving. Throughout our history inept problem solvers have created at least two problems for every one they think they have solved. Current problem solving is usually nothing more than a rearrangement of the variables. Doing this confuses the issues for a while, but solves nothing and leads to us having to deal with a nefarious jungle of bad problem solving on top of other bad problem solving. Just imagine if you had assumed that $7 \times 7 = 65$ and then made some decisions based on that, and still more decisions based on those, and so on. That, folks, is essentially where we are today.

> "The significant problems we face cannot be solved at the same level of thinking we were at when we created them."
> – Albert Einstein

To elucidate this with a contemporary problem, let's say that a fifty-year-old man is told by his doctor that he has high cholesterol. The doctor prescribes the "solution"– cholesterol-lowering drugs. Is this really the solution to the problem? Firstly, even the television commercials that tout these drugs often make the disclaimer that they may not reduce the incidence of heart attacks, which is supposedly the reason we need to lower our cholesterol. Secondly, taking these drugs allows the man to continue living the same lifestyle that is causing the root problem, albeit with an artificial reduction in cholesterol levels. Millions of people are on these medications, and yet over one million people a year die from heart disease in the United States alone. So taking these pills gives the man a temporary illusion that his problem is solved, until his first heart attack – or his last.

Notwithstanding any myopic benefit, where do you suppose all these medical concoctions end up after millions of these drug takers go to the toilet? The world's water is being tainted by people thinking they're solving a problem. Such tainted water does (and will) create more problems than we can possibly foresee. Therefore, solving this problem incorrectly is really no solution at all and actually creates even more problems. Thirty years from now people will be getting strange diseases from tainted drinking water. Will they be able to easily identify that it was from all the medications their meat-eating parents were gulping? Let's learn to solve problems correctly now, because thirty years from now there will only be more layers of problems concealing the real solution.

Still other personal and societal problems flourish and multiply because people *choose* to believe that cholesterol-lowering drugs solve problems, then base more decisions on bad solutions. Denial and hypocrisy are interwoven into such a lifestyle and are still more problematic. If you care to become a true problem solver, you will encounter massive hypocrisy and denial, some of it your own. Acknowledge it, see it for what it is, reject it and move past it. Hypocrisy and denial have no place in real solutions.

Yikes.

Consider an example of an oak tree that represents a given problem. A little ant sitting atop this mighty oak might have difficulty understanding that a branch on one side of the tree is connected to another branch on the other side of the tree. Nonetheless, the pathway leading up by way of dozens and dozens of divergences, forks in the road, if you will, is also, were the ant to turn around, a pathway down by way of convergences of those forks. As the ant finds the pathway down, he can see where smaller, seemingly unrelated branches come together. At each convergence of branches there is a small solution to small problems and a glimpse into further insights ahead. Continuing down, the larger branches converge, creating greater and greater solutions and insight. The trunk awaits those few ants that make the entire journey.

If an ant was on a branch on the left side of the tree and wanted to be on a branch on the right side of the tree, it _must_ go back to the convergence of branches that would allow for that particular change in direction. If, instead of going back to that convergence, the ant continued moving up, believing that "something" would get him there (a strong wind, perhaps), he would only succeed in confusing the issue (and himself) and getting farther from where he really wants to be.

Fortunately, any path that leads up can also lead back. Unfortunately, most people follow the path up, thinking this is progress. It is only progress insofar as it is the progression of problems, not the solving of them. If you want real solutions, you first need to go back to from where they emanate. Only then can you know what changes need to be made in the plotting of your new course.

Step Back

It is often surprising to learn the real root of our problems. The process of problem solving can be long and painful, but the rewards are empowering and can be life altering – for the better. There is a method that can be utilized to find almost any solution you could possibly want, but the real solutions may be hard to accept. Part of problem solving is developing the desire to recognize *and* embrace the real solution – truth cuts both ways. Most people quickly skip over the wrongs they commit, yet are usually pretty harsh with others who do the same things. In becoming a true problem solver, you need to become your own harshest critic, and your own best friend. You should know that if properly guided, and with proper intention, abiding with suffering is the paradoxical way out.

> *"Whoso loveth knowledge loveth correction; but he that is brutish hateth reproof."* – Proverbs 12:14

This process of problem solving is called "stepping back." It is very similar to the physical process of the ant going back to find the trunk, except this is a mental process. Stepping back actually refers to the thought process of coming to a given problem and then considering from where that problem originally came. It takes the development of this skill, complete truth to oneself and a complete abandonment of one's "wants" to be able to decipher the real predecessor of the original problem. As you develop this skill – and art – you should be able to step back one further to the preceding problem. Rinse and repeat until you get to the real root of the problem. In mathematics, they call this finding the common denominator. Many problems (even seemingly unrelated ones) have the same common denominator, or cause.

Stepping back can be aptly thought of as an individual's pursuit of truth, and you can take it as far as you want to, all the way to the source, if you so desire. Give yourself some quiet time to try it. Contrary to popular practice, wherein loud debate reigns supreme, it is in quiet time with oneself that answers can be found.

One of the possible traps of stepping back is known in Latin as "post hoc, ergo propter hoc," which literally means "after this, therefore because of this." This term is often used in economics to illustrate a fallacy and caution against an incorrect flow of assumptions. For example, if interest rates were reduced on Monday and more jobs were created on Tuesday, one might make the assumption that lower interest rates caused the increase in jobs. More thought is necessary to determine whether this is, in fact, true. It could be that the increase in jobs on Tuesday was caused by the weather or any number of other variables that have nothing to do with interest rates.

So let's try to use this method on that same fifty-year-old man at risk of a heart attack. The problem seemingly at hand is high cholesterol, but let's step back to see where his high cholesterol is coming from. Cholesterol is a fatty substance found in animals, but it is nonexistent in plants. Therefore, this man's high cholesterol is actually coming from the animal products he is ingesting. Vegans, obviously, are usually found to have dramatically lower levels of cholesterol than meat eaters. So surely, in order to eliminate the problem of high cholesterol, wouldn't it make sense to eliminate the animal products from his diet rather than pump him full of drugs? To do otherwise would be like trying to solve the problem of drunk driving by developing a pill that helps you pass a Breathalyzer test after ten martinis.

Meat eaters often have high cholesterol. Vegans almost never have high cholesterol. In fact, some doctors are now telling their patients to eat less meat and more vegetables. Part of this problem is that "less" meat isn't good enough. Now we have people who think they've improved their diet and still have high cholesterol, which contributes to their frustration and confusion. The solution is simple. Eliminate animal products. You will not get high cholesterol from eating too many carrots. Even though there is a vast array of vegan foods that offer a satisfying and healthy diet, many people may not like the solution, so they take statins and other drugs and the problem marches on – away from paradise.

Don't get mad at me, I warned you.

As you become more experienced with stepping back, you will find everything is connected. For many people, this concept is difficult to imagine. Virtually all schools teach us that there is an Atlantic Ocean, a Pacific Ocean, an Indian Ocean and so on. But the truth is *all* water is connected. Planet Earth has but one ocean. We drink from it, bathe in it and dump into it.

While naming bodies of water may, at first glance, help you understand where the gallons are located, it can be a far greater disservice to instill a separatist belief, because that leads to a philosophy of disconnection. This "education" is replete with truth-blocking misinformation. This teaching process would be better called a dis-education, and possibly an outright corruption. All water is connected, and all the Earth is connected.

Dis-education creates chasms between people who study ethics and morality, and those who utilize pragmatics and logic. Both sides often agree that ethics isn't necessarily logical. They're both wrong. There is always a pathway. Sometimes people can't see the path, but that doesn't mean it doesn't exist.

Finding the real answers, finding truth, is many things. First, it is painful, then curative and then rapturous. This process is enlightenment and, in a grander sense, it is love. In stepping back, you will know when you've reached the source because it is like being in love; you know it when you're there.

Go To The Source

A powerful tool in problem solving is to go back to the source of the original problem and then, having witnessed from where it actually emanates, you can change direction to bring about the desired solution.

There are an unlimited number of ways to visualize this process. One I have found to be most lucid is imagining the pipes of a plumbing system. Let's say you go to the faucet and turn it on but the water only trickles out. The problem is: No water. You go to a second faucet and turn it on and, again, only a trickle. You try a third faucet, but this time water flows out as it should. If you were able to climb into the first faucet and wiggle your way through the maze of pipes, eventually you would come to a convergence of two pipes (remember, you're going backwards toward the source, stepping back). At this junction, you see that there is no water. One of the pipes leads back from where you came, and one of the pipes leads to the second faucet you tried. Turn up toward the second faucet and you establish that this is not the source of the problem nor is it the area holding the solution. You need to step back again and continue moving toward the source.

Continue down your original pipe toward where you think there is another convergence, but you can't quite get there; it's blocked. Dig your way through the obstruction and, suddenly, water gushes toward you. You know you are facing the source, because it hits you in the kisser, not the back of the head. You have found the problem, you have cross-checked and you can now see why the faucets were dry. You see the source, and you see the water flowing properly to correct the drought. You have been enlightened.

If you hadn't pursued the solution correctly, you might have just sat back and thought that the city was out of water. You would have waited and waited and waited, assuming the water would come back on once "they" fixed the problem. Or you might simply have thought that your faucets were broken. Changing faucets would yield a bill from the hardware store but no water. However, you went to the source, found the real problem and solved it.

Stepping back can not only be used to find personal solutions, it can be thought of as the pursuit of larger and larger truths. Knowing when you're at an intersection is easy, like the ant on the oak tree coming to a convergence of branches or your microscopic self at a junction of pipes in your home's water supply, but how do you know which is the correct route to take?

Go Beyond Ten Percent

Fortunately for us humans, we have a brain. Learn how to use it.

Schools and universities the world over teach people to follow their misdirection more than they do to think (problem # 57,946,493,939). Case in point: We now have doctors, some of society's most highly "educated" problem solvers, addressing high cholesterol and obesity with statin drugs and surgery.

Not coincidentally, it is said we only use ten percent of our brain. Certainly this has been hotly debated, and probably to the largest extent by the offended ten-percenters. Whether the number is five percent, ten percent, twenty percent or more, the point is the same. We don't have to dive into a plumbing system and, by trial and error, try to get to a given destination. We can lay out road maps in our minds, test every single avenue to see where it leads, retract as necessary, and proceed on to the next. And the next, and the next. Become an adventurer, an experimenter, and a witness to all possibilities – become a thinker. As you step back from a given problem and come to a convergence, you will now be in a position to explore where those forks lead. Use truth and hypocrisy as litmus tests. You must embrace truth, as this is the problem solver's tool. You must personally abandon denial and hypocrisy, the problem solver's nemeses.

Sadly, in today's world most people never question mutually exclusive thoughts, such as having a belief that killing is wrong but that there is nothing wrong with eating hamburgers. The way most people live and "think" is confusing, truth-blocking, troublesome, dysfunctional, problematic and even somewhat schizoid.

> *"There's a schizoid quality to our relationship with animals, in which sentiment and brutality exist side by side. Half the dogs in America will receive Christmas presents this year, yet few of us pause to consider the miserable life of the pig – an animal easily as intelligent as a dog – that becomes the Christmas ham."*
> – "An Animal's Place," by Michael Pollan,
> *New York Times Magazine*, Nov. 10, 2002

Welcome truth and reject hypocrisy wherever they are found. By doing so, stepping back can be used to fix the plumbing problems in your house or city. Stepping back can be used to fix personal and marital problems. Stepping back can be used to fix societal and planetary problems. This method can help you get beyond your own circumstances, to see outside yourself, to see not only the trees but the forest as well. To see past our own individual set of circumstances is essential in finding real solutions.

As you develop the stepping back method to problem solving, you may very well generate thousands of "pipes" that are seemingly unrelated. Draw it out on paper if you need to, but it is important that you use your brain. Think. As small pipes lead into larger pipes, and those pipes lead into still larger pipes, you will begin to see that problems have common denominators. Perhaps, even, a single common denominator. You will actually use your brain in the process, and probably far more than ten percent of it. Plus, the more you think, the more insight you will garner, and the more insight you garner, the more you can think.

Wisdom lies in wait for those, and only those, who endeavor to find it. Wisdom is not a birthright, it is an accomplishment born of years of hard and properly guided work.

"What wisdom can you find that is greater than kindness?"
                                                    – Pierre Rousseau

The chapters in this book are each like a water main. Every one outlines a problem and then steps back to its solution. Though seemingly unrelated at first, the chapters are all connected and you will see that each solution is the same solution.

There is a solitary answer, a truth, that can solve almost all of our problems, because almost all of our problems stem from the same cause. Thousands of years ago, the Garden of Eden was a paradise, and it fell from paradise due to one cataclysmic event, changing man's existence on Planet Earth. That event was said to be eating the forbidden fruit. But it was not an apple or a fig. In fact, it was not a fruit at all.

Solving almost all of our problems by locating and correcting the one root cause would actually be quite simple if it weren't for one thing; it is now also the forbidden truth. I will get you to that source, where the answer is clear: Veganism for all mankind. What you do once at the source, align yourself with it or deny it, is up to you.

To be perfectly clear, veganism in and of itself cannot automatically solve every problem on the planet. You can be vegan but still be a liar. But without veganism, our real problems cannot truly be solved. Embracing the principles of veganism assures all solutions. Veganism is the foundation upon which a true civilization must be built.

Whereas religious leaders may condone eating meat and then tell us to put some money in the collection cup, God wants you to be vegan. "Thou Shalt Not Kill." If you believe it but don't live it, we've all got a problem.

This book will help you solve it.

Chapter 2

Truth

"This above all, to thy own self be true.
And it must follow as the night the day;
Thou canst not then be false to anyone."
                    – *Hamlet,* by William Shakespeare

Deceiving other people is bad. Deceiving yourself is a tragedy. If you spend some money but then tell your spouse that you didn't, you are creating blockages to truth. If you spend money but then tell *yourself* that you didn't, you're up the creek without a paddle. How can you even hope to tell others the truth? How would you know the truth? Recognizing truth becomes impossible and, therefore, abstract. But truth is not abstract.

If you would like to live in a paradise, your actions need to reflect that decision. For example, in a paradise truth would prevail over deception. The very first lie you tell, no matter how little or white it may be, begins to detract from the paradise that *you've* chosen. Moreover, if each person on the planet (over six billion now) chose to live in a paradise and then told one little white lie, there would be over six billion lies told. That's a lot of deception – and paradise dissipates. Of course, no one is perfect. In fact, you should shun concepts of perfection and instead pursue excellence. Every time you speak, whether to others or, even more importantly, to yourself, you have an opportunity to create excellence in truthfulness.

You also have an opportunity to create something less than excellence with deception. Deception operates as tangibly as a veil blocks light, and today there are numerous veils obscuring paradise. For example, faith is necessary for those who choose paradise, believe in God and yet refuse to live their lives accordingly. Faith would not be necessary if the veil were removed. Veils can be removed by your actions, my actions and everyone's actions. Truth, love and many of the other splendid elements of paradise, perhaps even God, would be omnipresent – no faith required.

> *"Blessed are the pure in heart: for they shall see God."*
> – Matthew 5:8

Let's say that we all choose paradise and live our lives accordingly. We're truthful, loving, humanitarian, caring and so on. And let's say that once we've put all this into place God still does not reveal Himself. What are we left with? Paradise. We have, in effect, created a Godlike existence upon this planet without a need for Him to prove His existence. The lesson here is that each behavior you need to use to create paradise stands on its own merit, and each utilized together lifts the veil more and more. Do not allow those people who create veils convince you that nothing is behind them.

This may seem a bit abstract, so allow me to use a tangible example. As you take the first step on a ladder your horizon increases. Each step up gives you a better vista. This is an absolute fact. What views await you? You'll have to climb up to see. I told you earlier, you will have to do your part. If you choose to be mindful, loving, caring, humanitarian and truthful, and then educate and inspire others to be the same, and they in turn continue this process with still others, would not the world truly be so much better? This is a paradise in the making. Don't let the abstract philosophy get in the way of the tangible and logical betterment for yourself, others and the world around you. It need not be any more complex than simply understanding that when you step up a ladder you are higher than before. Also understand that before you can see the vista from step number two you need to get to step number one.

Deceit is a veil, and it operates as a roadblock on the road to paradise. What's more, deceit is problematic, creating more roadblocks. The asphalt continues, but you have been blocked, and blockages tend to create bigger blockages. Then, those who attempt to justify their misguided lifestyle try to convince you that nothing lies beyond the roadblock. Enough blocked people converge and all agree, which tends to convince still others. The other side of the roadblock becomes abstract. But it isn't. Strive to do all you can to remove the roadblocks from your daily behavior. It will help others to do the same. Pursue truth.

You can claim to be virtuous, loving, humanitarian, spiritual, pious, healthy and even truthful without being vegan, but it would all be a lie. The words "deceit" and "insidious" have close etymological ties. Clearly, deceit begins an insidious process that takes us away from the place we want to be. Deceit is one blockage, and the key to lifting all blockages is being vegan. Veganism also allows for the complete removal of hypocrisy, which is another blockage of truth. If you're like me, you consider yourself to be an animal lover. If you're like I was before I became vegan, you eat animal flesh. That is blockage-causing hypocrisy. Veganism is the common thread that weaves together all genuine virtue sans hypocrisy.

Clarity In Truth

Unfortunately, the word "truth" is every bit as misunderstood as the word "vegan." I have serious concerns that this is far from coincidence. In fact, veganism and truth go hand in hand. Conversely, meat and deception are one and the same. Even the word "meat" is a deception. It's flesh, folks.

The word truth, as it is commonly used, refers to the conveyance of information believed to be factual from one person to another. For example, your mother believes that milk is good for you, so she tells you to drink it. Unfortunately, this is nothing more than a subjective truth. This is a belief that has been passed down from generation to generation but has no basis in truth at all.

A distinction should be made between truth and honesty. A mother telling her child that milk is good for him or her is being honest, because she believes what she is saying to be true. But cow's milk, as you will learn later, is not good for humans. Therefore, this mother is not being truthful, albeit unintentionally. It is a sad and troubling reality that we have a world where there is little honesty and far less truth.

"Truth is not hard to kill," but "… a lie well told is immortal." —*Advice to Youth*, Mark Twain

Hidden beneath the many layers of the many subjective "truths" in our world lies objective, or real, truth. You can call it objective truth, real truth, divine truth, natural truth, but it is simply truth. Truth does not come from ego, desire, politics, subjectivity, indoctrination, tradition or custom. Nor does it change in order to win friends, enhance careers, make money, accumulate power or sell more milk. So, you might ask, what is truth and where does it come from? The short answer is that truth is fact, and fact reveals itself when veils are lifted. But if you speak untruths (to yourself or others), even just to win friends or enhance careers, truth disappears, and then you'll have to ask again, "What is truth and where does it come from?"

Given the world's current condition, truth is not necessarily quick or easy, but if you choose paradise, it is the only ticket.

Meat And The Big Lie

People in our society who want (desire) to eat meat pass laws (politics) to say it is perfectly okay (subjectivity). They then teach (indoctrination) children to eat meat (tradition), and the entire process perpetuates itself with each new generation (custom). I call this process The Big Lie.

Unfortunately, the timelessness of The Big Lie clouds truth to such an extent that truth is now all but impossible to see. The Big Lie has led us all up the creek. Not coincidentally, even the concept of truth itself can seem subjective and abstract. In a crazy world, it is the sane man who looks crazy. Most attempts to discuss truth with people who can't see past their subjective truth will yield responses such as, "Truth? Whose truth?" or "Your truth isn't my truth." We now have a society that views truth subjectively and its misguided lifestyle as objectively proper.

> *"Mere precedent is a dangerous source of authority."*
> – Andrew Jackson

The democratic process reinforces this ever-increasing distance from truth. Democracy embraces debate and majority rule, but what do semantics and numbers have to do with truth? Belief in debate gives life to the fallacy that putting words in a poetic or semantically correct order means those words are correct. Belief in majority rule is the very genesis of might over right. Both of these beliefs offer nothing of truth.

This is not meant to be an indictment of the democratic process. In fact, democracy is better than any other system in place at the moment. But better doesn't mean good. A good and decent society, worthy of being labeled civilized, must be based on truth. Truth is truth, whether a lot of people embrace it or just one person or no people at all, for that matter. Remember that water is wet whether you live on the beach or in the desert. Truth is truth, whether stentorian or tacit. Truth is truth whether it sounds appealing or not.

> *"If observance to Truth were a bed of roses, if Truth cost one nothing and were all happiness and ease, there would be no beauty about it. We must adhere to Truth even if the heavens should fall."*   – Mahatma Gandhi

Sadly, lies can be made to seem more appealing than truth. For example, McDonald's showing off their smiling hamburgers has done more to malign truth than perhaps any other commercial venture in the history of the world. Truth: Hamburgers and chicken nuggets come from immense suffering – and cause even more suffering.

> *"O Disciples, know this: eventually, impostors will appear everywhere, deceiving the people and teaching them that they can devour meat and still attain enlightenment and salvation."*   – The Buddha

Society is becoming increasingly violent, diseased and dystopian because we are clinging more and more to subjective truth. People are telling themselves lies. So call it what you will – subjective truth, propaganda, political truth, a silly belief or call it what it really is, a Big Lie – it is carrying Planet Earth away from truth and paradise at the speed of light.

The Big Lie is preventing you from seeing what's on the other side of the veil. If you choose utopia over dystopia, tell yourself truth and only truth, and then speak it to others.

Granted, turning one's back on indoctrination, on subjective truth, on The Big Lie, is no small task. Truth is the much less traveled road. But the rewards of the stepping back journey are magnificent beyond all that glitters. Make the choice to open your mind and your heart to what is true. You will discover concepts you never considered before, or even knew existed. Be warned. Others will try to pull you back onto the subjective expressway, but ask yourself if what you believe is true or if you just want it to be true. The latter offers a degree of familiarity and seeming comfort, but is not necessarily truth. Forge on and ask yourself the hard questions. This may seem a paradox, but it is the only road to paradise.

While it is immensely sad to consider that what most people in today's world seek most is to have their way be true, it is tremendously empowering and enlightening to change this pattern in ourselves. Rather than spend your life seeking your way to be true, seek truth most of all and have it be your way. This is the practical and literal difference between good and evil, enlightenment and darkness.

As you proceed, you will find yourself becoming true with yourself, true with all those around you, and you'll find yourself becoming vegan. The darkness of confusion and turmoil are eradicated in truth's brilliant light. Further, truth breeds harmony, and harmony is the essence of veganism. They are intertwined.

Speak only truth, even if it's only to yourself at first, in order to realize ever-increasing and more vivid truth. It is very much like a blurred picture that slowly comes into focus. Even if, right now, you choose to be completely truthful henceforth, it will still take time. There is no sudden arrival of truth. It is achieved through long, hard work. (The same goes for enlightenment, love, wisdom, humanity, peace, etc. – the many attributes of paradise we will be discussing.)

Imagine that you are the proverbial one-hundred-pound weakling. You decide right now that you want to be a big, strong bodybuilder. The moment of that decision can set into motion a new lifestyle, but you are still a one-hundred-pound weakling. You begin eating right and going to the gym regularly. But even after each grueling workout, there is virtually no appreciable difference in your strength or appearance. It is only after many workouts over a long period of time that there can be a sudden recognition of how much you've changed. The process of getting to that recognition is long and arduous, and more rewarding than winning the lottery. Personal empowerment is on a different plateau from random gain. There is nothing more rewarding than choosing paradise and doing your part to effect it. It will help others do the same, and when enough people unite under the principles of paradise, it will facilitate not a sudden arrival, but a sudden realization of what was a challenging task.

Choose truth, live in harmony and be vegan, as these are one and the same, and you will help to create the paradise on Earth that nature originally intended.

The Rules Of The Game

Every game you play, whether it is Monopoly, Scrabble or a simple game of cards, has a set of rules. For the duration of the game these rules are truth, if you will. So let's not make truth a mystical thing. Some can claim that paradise doesn't exist or never will exist. But as you and I and others embrace truth and use truth, the picture of paradise gets clearer. In simple and practical terms, truth is the rulebook on how to achieve life in the paradise we've chosen. If you want to live in paradise and, therefore, create harmony for all, you must behave by certain rules. Truth, by design, gives us those rules, whereas the lack of it, also by design, takes us away from paradise and into dystopia.

Truth can also aptly be thought of as a technical tool used to connect to other truths that connect to still more truths. With proper usage, this technical tool can actually get us to a fundamental reality. So no matter what medical research may claim is "healthy," killing and eating animals is violent, removes harmony for all and obliterates paradise. Ever-increasing truth offers ever-increasing clarity. This is the only path to the health we all seek.

Seek truth, align yourself with it, and help us all to achieve our paradise. Hey, maybe we'll call this place VeganWorld.

Chapter 3

The Defining Moment

I can't count the number of vegetarians I run into who tell me they eat a little bit of chicken and fish now and then. As a result, it is important to precisely define some of the words and concepts we will be discussing.

Meat: Meat is any and all animal flesh. Some people think "meat" means beef. No. Beef means beef. Meat *can* mean beef, but meat also means chicken, raccoon, fish, elephant, cockroach, lobster, aardvark, turkey, dolphin, ostrich, rabbit, eagle, man, frog, cat, zebra, clam, alligator, dog, giraffe, etc. Meat is simply a generic term for the flesh of any animal.

Vegetarian: One who eats no meat. Vegetarians mostly eat plant-based foods, though some animal products, such as eggs and dairy, may be included in their diet. Eating eggs and dairy products still qualifies as being vegetarian because milk, cheese, yogurt and eggs, etc., can be produced without killing animals, at least in theory. (The practical truth is another story entirely, which we will get into later.) Vegetarians may also abstain from products that are produced by killing an animal, such as leather, fur and many soaps and beauty products. A vegetarian may use wool, which, again, at least theoretically, can be produced without harming sheep.

Vegan: (Pronounced VEE-gan, with the accent on the first syllable and then a hard "g".) One who consumes no meat, dairy or animal products of any kind whatsoever. Vegans wear no animal products, such as leather or fur, nor use products made from or tested on animals. Vegans typically believe that animals are not on this planet for human exploitation of any kind – food, clothing, entertainment, experimentation, etc. Veganism holds that simply because animals can't speak English (or Spanish or Chinese or Russian) is not a valid reason to exploit them.

"Dietary vegans" are people who eat a vegan diet but may use other types of animal products. In a meat-producing world, it can sometimes be quite a challenge at first to completely eliminate all animal products, and it should be understood that becoming vegan is a process – the pursuit of excellence, not perfection. If you pursue excellence enough, you won't need to engage in the folly of questioning whether or not you'll arrive there. Nonetheless, as in any practical application, there is a complete spectrum, but the philosophy and definition of veganism remains as an absolute and an ideal.

"Ethical vegans" are those who make the choice to be vegan irrespective of health benefits.

Those of you who have been paying attention will have noticed that there is a glaring omission from the list of definitions above. As of this writing, it is a concept so widely understood and accepted that there isn't even a word for it. One who does *not* eat any animal products is, as you now know, called a vegan. One who *does* eat flesh and animal products is called a _____. The answer is … Sorry, I don't know either. We don't publicly call vegans "herbivores," so I suppose we can rule out calling meat eaters "carnivores." Mr. Webster, where are you when I need you?

Well, yes, I guess you could call them meat eaters, but as I see it, that would be improper. The word "meat" is just a construct to put distance between what you are really eating and what you want to think you are eating. Throughout the ages, and even in the Bible, the word meat has sometimes been used metaphorically to simply mean food. But meat, I mean flesh, I mean meat – you know what I mean – is not food. "Meat" just doesn't sound quite as grotesque as "flesh." Flesh eater would be more accurate, but somewhat repulsive sounding, so I doubt that it would be widely adopted. The fact that it is accurate *and* repulsive should tell us something about those who partake of animal flesh and choose to call it meat.

Well, geez, does anyone have a suggestion?

Let's Call A Spade A Spade

Remarkably, those who eat absolutely anything and everything, no matter how repulsive, unhealthy, cruel, environmentally hazardous or blasphemous, are considered so normal and mainstream that they are in no need of categorization. In truth, however, it is impossible to have a healthy, decent, civilized society while nothing healthy, decent or civilized is embraced by that society. Conversely, those who eat healthily, care for themselves and others, including animals, live in harmony with the environment and nature, and walk along the path of God are labeled with a "V" word. "Hey, you, vegan. Go stand over there."

Society's current penchant for subjective truth, for The Big Lie, in which meat eaters have no label, would be replaced by truth if more people embraced veganism. In such a new era of truth and harmony, meat might be called flesh, and flesh would be seen as a product of violence. After all, what is more violent than killing? What is considered normal and mainstream today would be considered repulsive, cruel, barbaric and even criminal, as might over right is a necessary tool of the flesh eater. The indefinable

majority today would have to whisper under their breath
that they eat animals. In fact, from a platform of truth, I
think it would be very easy to find a label for these people. As
society moves toward veganism, it will become "normal" to
be vegan. No need for a label. The word "normal" will not be
defined solely by the number of participants, as it is now, but
by society's alignment with truth.

   Interestingly, the word "normal" has connotations of
correctness or of being right. This is as it _should_ be. The
problem comes when normalcy is defined by subjective
truth, as it is today. To illustrate this point, consider that in
Nazi Germany it was normal to be racist. But was normalcy
based upon subjective truth or real truth? The Nazis wanted
their subjective truth to be true. This is part of what made
Nazi Germany evil. They waged world war, engaged in
genocide and pursued the absurd notion of a superior race,
all because of a belief that was nothing more than a
subjective truth or, to be accurate, an outright lie. Even if the
Nazis had prevailed and now ruled the world, their beliefs
would still not be true. No act of man, no matter how great
or infamous, could ever make this desire for control a truth.

> _"The time will come when men such as I will look upon
> the murder of animals as they now look upon the
> murder of men."_   – Leonardo da Vinci

Chicken (the meat) is actually chicken (the bird). We
currently murder about ten billion (yes, 10,000,000,000)
animals every year, and that figure doesn't even include fish
and other ocean animals. Can meat possibly be reconciled
with peace, love and harmony on a ledger of truth? Even
meat from one animal is deceit, violence and murder, let
alone from ten billion.

> _9.8 billion birds and mammals were bred and killed for
> food in the U.S._ – Latest annual calculation, United
> States Department of Agriculture

Can harmony for all exist while society eats meat? Of course not. Can harmony for any exist while society eats meat? Can we progress on the road to paradise while society eats meat? Though it may be hard to admit out loud, you know the answer.

When A Heart Is A Heart

The bottom line is always the same when you use truth as a ledger. Veganism is about truth, love, empathy and compassion, from which individual and environmental health flourish. As a result, society and all its parts will benefit manifold as each of us becomes vegan. In this vegan society it will be normal to be vegan, and this normalcy will be based on truth. My hope is that it will also be based on numbers.

When this day is finally upon us, it will be interesting to see who remembers the fact that we were once all criminals. Indeed, part of the pain and subsequent joy we experience as we become vegan is to remember how far we've each moved forward, and to recognize from where we each have come.

"The greatness of a nation can be judged by the way its animals are treated."   – Mahatma Gandhi

Chapter 4

Love

"There is only misfortune in not being loved; there is misery in not loving."   – Albert Camus

Everybody knows what love is, right? Perhaps. All people are born with the ability to love, as we all innately possess that emotion. Unfortunately, however, most people never learn how to properly express love. Did you ever take a class in "How to love?" Forget majoring in it, just one basic class? Even as children grow into adults, I think it's safe to say all people know the emotion of love. But love is far, far more than an emotion. It is a behavior. The emotion is the tool, whereas the behavior is the application, or use, of the tool. Owning a wrench, for example, is pointless unless you know how to use it – and then use it. Sadly, most people never learn the practical application of love, and therein lies a very, very, very large problem.

It is critically important for one's own growth to understand that *all* people spend their lives in pursuit of the *exact same thing* – love. It is important to understand this basic principle, because doing so can help to remove the elements of separatism and hatred from how we lead our lives and replace them with a sense of personal responsibility, forgiveness, understanding and an increased ability to accept and love all others. From this platform, you will understand that the bully in school possesses the emotion of love as much as the nice kid he's bullying. The man who beats up his wife every other Monday loves her just as much as the man who sends his wife flowers every other Tuesday. Members of a street gang and members of a church choir make very different sounds, but possess the very same quantity of love. Even Adolf Hitler and Mahatma Gandhi, the seemingly oddest of couples, were both on a similar course, looking for the very same thing – love. Come to think of it, this may very well be the first book ever written that included Adolf Hitler in a chapter about love. It's about time. Maybe now we'll get somewhere. The objective here is not to offend, but to elucidate truth. Truth must be pursued and embraced, even if it hurts.

Everyone wants the exact same thing because we are all equipped the exact same way. We all have the same tools: we all have a heart, we all have a brain and we all have emotions. To use an analogy, all Corvettes possess the exact same equipment. While 'Vettes are nice to look at and fun to drive, some Corvettes might be used in bank robberies whereas some might be used to deliver food to the hungry. Clearly, it's all in how the equipment is used. Good and evil are far more than ethereal concepts, they are actions. Maybe some more definitions are in order.

Good And Evil

The word "evil" can conjure up images of a red guy with horns. This may lead some to believe that if you aren't red with horns then you must not be evil. This is a very dangerous, though widely accepted, notion. No matter what the physical form, evil is a behavior – with or without red horns. If there were a red guy with horns who only did good and loving deeds, would he be evil? Similarly, the word "good" also refers to a behavior. We can accurately say that one who engages in evil behavior is evil and one who engages in good behavior is good.

Webster's New World Dictionary defines evil as "wicked, depraved, causing pain or trouble; harmful; injurious." Remember this definition anytime you hear the word "meat" or "flesh." The same dictionary offers a lengthy list of words to define the word "good," some of which are "pleasant, healthy, honorable, right, kind, virtuous, pious, sympathetic." Again, remember this definition anytime you hear the word "meat" or "flesh" and ask yourself if it applies. Then remember the word "vegan."

People who become vegan for the purpose of losing weight or correcting a disease may very well accomplish their goal, but often encounter willpower issues, whereas people who understand good and evil can become vegan without ever looking back. Once you understand the teams, it's simply a matter of asking yourself on which side you want to be.

Since the majority of people in the world believe in God, I'll put it like this: We were *all* created in God's image, not just some of us. We all possess the emotion of love – the tool – and, innately, we want the exact same thing, to experience that emotion. How we learn to express that emotion, or use the tool, however, is the difference between good and evil. People learn love and its expression in many different ways, and the difference is as stark as Adolf Hitler and Mahatma Gandhi. The proper application of love is the very connection to God, whereas the lack of it is the disconnection.

It is an outright indictment on our society and education systems that most people learn the application of love through random rites of passage. While reading, writing and arithmetic are vitally important, the stepping back process also helps us to recognize priorities. Love is more important than calculus, and yet by the time children are being taught calculus, not one class has been offered to them on how to love. To make matters worse, all we have as a role model is a violent, dysfunctional world. Some people pick up on more of that dysfunction than others, but it really is no more than a violence lottery. It should be obvious, therefore, that it is critically important to learn how to apply the emotion of love as a behavior. Learn how to *use* the tool.

> *"The most momentous thing in human life is the art of winning the soul to good or to evil."*   – Pythagoras

Two more words must be elucidated here in the same section where we discuss evil. The first is the word "hypocrisy." *Webster's New World Dictionary* defines hypocrisy as "pretending to be what one is not, or to feel what one does not feel; especially a pretense of virtue, piety, etc." If love is "good," can love and hypocrisy coexist? Can you truly believe "Thou shalt not kill" and then go have a hamburger?

This brings up the second word: "Denial." On second thought, I'll leave that one alone. We all know what it means.

The Golden Rule

Evil and hypocrisy can be replaced by the proper application of love, and applying love as a behavior is the very key to changing the world. As individuals learn to express love properly, the synergistic effect on the world will be grand. Love as an action is as simple as treating others as you would want all others to treat you. These are words thrown around like a Frisbee, but the real lesson is much harder to learn. Yet this is the lesson most people need to learn, because when you do you can no longer beat up others, wage world war in the name of superiority or abuse animals. (Yes, folks, eating animals is abuse.)

Within the execution of proper love there is an understanding that we all long for the very same thing – love. Within proper love there is empathy and an understanding that love is a service *to* others, not an expectation *from* others. And at the core of the proper application of love is veganism. Within proper love there is no hypocrisy.

Don't Blame Adolf

It should go without saying that a society that embraces authority contains a certain degree of dementia. It is a time bomb waiting to happen. The fuse is lit when one of the leading demented minds is given power to rule. Moreover, when a sociopath is given the power to rule, those endowing him with that power need a thorough mental examination as much as the sociopath. There's a huge lesson here; maybe more than one.

Meat And The Sociopath

An understanding of what constitutes a sociopath will shed even more light on the subject of love. It can be said that sociopaths are missing something. Just as a blind man is missing his sight, a sociopath is missing his ability to commune with humanity. Sociopaths can *seem* otherwise, but they are actually antisocial. A primary trait of sociopaths is that they don't feel the pain of others, only their own. It is a chilling thought to know there are people out there who can't grasp empathy. After all, empathy is a fundamental part of humanity. Yet even more chilling is the fact that we have become a society of sociopaths. Harsh? Perhaps. But truth does not allow for the mincing of words.

Loving your mother but refusing to acknowledge that cows or dogs want that same opportunity is sociopathic. When we look at the tiny microcosm known as our family, we understand the sacred bond that exists between its members. Yet, by eating meat and dairy, we deny others that sacred bond. Do baby chickens, for example, not love their mothers? They follow them around like they're still attached. Be it people, cows, chickens or any other animal, brothers love brothers. To eat an animal is to kill someone's family member and selfishly deny them that same love we know is sacred. Eating meat and dairy is a roadblock to proper love. Moreover, in truth we are all family.

In a world of people who all claim to know the emotion of love, where are these sociopaths coming from? The answer to this question will be difficult to accept until such time as truth is seen as the goal rather than the search for blame. Be your own harshest critic for the purpose of being your own best friend.

The Big Lie is the main ingredient in creating meat eaters. In order for people to swallow the flesh of what was another living being, they must first learn to suppress innate empathy and, as just shown, not feeling empathy for other sentient creatures is the essence of a sociopath. Creating a world of meat eaters is creating a world of sociopaths. But *you* must choose truth and love as your tools if you want to break out of this cycle and progress on the path to paradise.

And while we're on the subject, let's just get this one out of the way. There are those who believe that animals are not sentient creatures, that they have no emotions or feelings. I can only assume that those people have never lived with a dog or cat or spent any time around animals. It takes about five minutes with a dog, for example, to see that they experience pain, pleasure, joy and excitement. Accidentally step on a dog's tail and it will yelp in pain. Do it intentionally and regularly, and the dog will learn to be nasty, like the person mistreating it. Scratch a cat's chin and it will purr in delight. Animals also dream, make conscious decisions and even sulk. Dogs, cats and parrots are no different from cows, pigs, chickens, fish or any of the other animals we commonly slaughter for food. Each and every one of those ten billion a year has a distinct personality, along with the same desire we all have – love. If you want paradise, choose truth. A sociopathic trait is to criticize cultures that eat dogs and then bite down on a hamburger.

The ability to deny the pain of another in one's mind is the very essence of eating animals. It is also the very essence of a sociopath. Now, I am not suggesting that all meat eaters are the same as Hitler (although there are billions of cows and pigs and fish who would), but I am saying that meat eaters and sociopaths utilize the very same psychological justifications. They are neither loving nor truthful. They have opaque veils before them. Not all people become icons of antisocial behavior, just as not all buildings are skyscrapers, but they are all made out of bricks, mortar and steel. A meat-eating society knows love only as an emotion, rather than as a behavior. The emotion of love tied to subjective truth and indoctrination produces bullies of every kind and magnitude. They only know *their* pain, and are lost in confusion while vainly chasing the love they crave.

Problems of every kind and magnitude are generated in a society of sociopaths, especially when sociopathic lifestyles are considered normal. According to a Zogby poll taken in 2000, more than ninety percent of the population eats meat, and it would be a fair assumption to say that practically all of them consider themselves good people who know what love is. From this "love" comes all the problems we see proliferating in our world today.

To the meat eater, the sociopath, animals must remain objects and products. But none of God's creatures are objects and products. That is as logical as suggesting it is okay to eat beef but not dog. All animals, including humans, are individuals with an absolute right to individual sovereignty and life. If you choose paradise, you must be truthful and loving. You must break out of the sociopathic way of meat eaters. You must acknowledge that eating meat causes pain to others. You must treat others as you would want to be treated. This is truth. This is love. This is vegan. This is the only road to paradise.

"But for the sake of some little mouthful of flesh, we deprive a soul of the sun and light and of that proportion of life and time it had been born into the world to enjoy."   – Plutarch

Stop The Evil Train

Because most children are innately empathetic, they love animals and would have nightmares if they witnessed an animal being hurt, particularly in the cruel and grotesque manner in which our meat industry slaughters. So when we first feed our children meat, do we show them pictures of the animal dying? No, of course not, because this would violate their innate compassion and empathy. Instead, we show them smiling hamburgers and dancing chicken nuggets. Then, once they have developed the taste for flesh, and the sociopathic methods are planted in their minds, any behavior can be justified for a lifetime.

"Custom will reconcile people to any atrocity."
                                    – George Bernard Shaw

Showing children pictures of, say, wheat being harvested is delightful and fun, yet when it comes to eating animals, we show them cartoon-like images of smiling meat products. Isn't that a lie? How can we endeavor to create a paradise when we lie to our youngest and most impressionable (creating future generations of liars)? Isn't this all a huge red flag to you? Teaching children it is perfectly okay to eat an animal begins the destruction of empathy and compassion and begins to lay the foundation for a lifetime of sociopathy. Clearly, we are systematically teaching children a very distorted and dysfunctional practice of love. We generate veils that block the children's view long before they even know what veils are. Children are then rendered virtually incapable of even recognizing the veils in front of them. They become adults who will do anything to justify their misguided wants and desires. In a word, sociopathic.

As children grow older, they embrace The Big Lie, which further clouds their innate empathy. The meat-eating society and its process works its insidious ways in their minds. Truth and empathy disappear. The proper application of love, which emanates from truth and empathy, is also gone. Our socio-pathic society now has children who proudly proclaim they love animals while eating a hamburger or a chicken nugget, and adults who can't figure out where all the violence is coming from.

This distortion of love is the fundamental stepping-stone to all brutality. And remember, brutality is nothing more than ill-learned love. Ill-learned love is replete with self-serving expectations *from* others rather than service *to* others. Ill-learned love is bullies, men who beat their wives *and* love them, and world leaders who start wars to make the world the way they want it because they believe it will bring them love (and is their way of giving love, believe it or not).

Well over ten billion animals are brutally murdered every year, and participation in this slaughter, in any capacity, is not proper love at all. It is sociopathic murder. However, meat eaters, being sociopaths, cannot see that eating animals is murder. Recognizing that would mean "loving, decent people" would have to stop the practice. But these "loving, decent people" want what they want. They don't want to know too much about the pain involved in producing their surf and turf. They only know their desire for it; hence, societal sociopathic murder under the pretense of love. But as for you, who choose paradise, you must also embrace truth – and speak it, at least to yourself for starters.

Serving meat to children is not proper love, for the server, the children or the animals. For the server, it is murder; for the children, it is child abuse; and for the animals, it is brutality.

Are You Ready For Love?

The only solution to the sociopathic insanity is to love in the proper manner; to use and implement love *as a behavior*. This proper love mandates that all mankind be vegan. In truth, the proper application of love would be to care for *all* others, and "all" includes animals that would otherwise be murdered. To truly implement love in our lives means to bestow upon all others the very behavior we would like bestowed upon us.

Sending out pretty greeting cards once a year extolling "Peace on Earth" and "Harmony for All" while eating an animal does nothing for peace or harmony. The difference between love as a behavior and love simply as an emotion is a key difference between good and evil.

> *"Though I speak with the tongues of men and angels, and have not love, I am become as sounding brass or a tinkling cymbal."* – 1 Corinthians 13:1

Proper love is so powerful in its effect that one chapter cannot fully elucidate its entire scope and range. This chapter gives you the basics, but every chapter in this book contains nuances of love that will help to give you the entire scope of what love really is – or should be. Some people refer to God as love. How powerful and far-reaching is that? It is interesting to consider that even in some of the most loving families, love exists only to a point – the boundaries of the family – and then it stops. Yet people look upon God's love as having no boundaries; after all, all of us on this fair planet are God's family. This should be telling us that if we want a loving, godly world, the love must extend to all – people and animals. Love that extends to all naturally mandates that meat be nonexistent.

The road to paradise is impassable when there is no proper love.

Chapter 5

Instinct

Webster's *New World Dictionary* defines instinct as "an inborn tendency to behave in a way characteristic of a species; natural unacquired mode of response to stimuli." In a natural realm, there is not a child on the planet who would try to murder an animal and eat it. The natural instinct of man tells us that we should not eat meat and that we should all be vegan. Unfortunately, The Big Lie and its processes do a magnificent job of tearing us from our instincts. When our natural instincts are corrupted and we begin to hunger for flesh, our society begins to crumble. If this misguided lifestyle is not quickly corrected, not only can we forget paradise, but we will ultimately be washed away by nature's current.

Don't Be Silly

The human instinct, being a product of nature, is a wonderful and powerful force to behold. Just think back to the first time you went fishing and you instinctively gasped at the horrid sight of the fish wriggling about with a hook in its mouth. Our dear fathers said to us what their fathers said to them: "Don't be silly. They don't feel it." Well, the truth is you weren't being silly then, so don't be silly now. OF COURSE THEY FEEL IT!

"If we believe absurdities, we shall commit atrocities."
                                                        – Voltaire

If fish, or any animal for that matter, could not feel pain (and pleasure) they could not possibly survive. If you didn't feel pain when you put your hands on a hot stove, you would burn your hands off. Without pain, you might never even know you lost your hands, at least until such time as your hunger pangs got the best of you and you tried to feed yourself. Oh, on second thought, what hunger pangs? You'd starve to death, happy as a lark.

Eating animals mandates that we quell our natural instincts of empathy, humanity and love, and spend our lives hiding from these attributes, which are the essence of humanity. Without the corruption of instinct and this ongoing denial, without the sociopathy, eating an animal would be impossible.

Too Close For Comfort

If you doubt that the natural instinct of human beings is to be vegan, put a baby in a crib with a rabbit and a carrot. Observe which one the child plays with and which one he eats. That is, until the parents tell the child to "try this." But even then, there's no way you'll get a child to eat the flesh of an animal if he knows what it is. Children are much closer to innate instinct and haven't yet been completely brainwashed by The Big Lie. To get a child to eat flesh, it must look like something else, at least until you have helped him develop a taste for it. Hamburgers, bologna sandwiches and chicken nuggets serve this purpose very well. Essentially, we must lie to children to get them to eat flesh, just as we lie to ourselves.

Even most adults who have eaten meat their whole lives and argue that man was meant to eat meat have a problem facing the reality of their inhumane practice. If, as they are chomping on a steak or a hot dog or a chicken sandwich, you ask them about the animal whose flesh they're eating, invariably the response comes, "Shut up. Can't you see I'm eating?" The brick wall of denial is very sturdy, and the flesh eater will quickly attempt to change the subject. The instincts may have been calloused by The Big Lie, but they're still there. Forge ahead with your questioning and the stress comes over them like a tropical rain. Conversely, try asking people who are eating fruit or vegetables about what it is they are consuming. The conversation will flow effortlessly, taking as many turns and shapes and colors as the plant foods they are eating. There is no stress generated when talking about how wheat is grown, harvested and prepared, even while eating a slice of bread.

You may have heard a meat eater say to a vegan, "Well, plants are alive, too. You shouldn't eat them, either." Of course, this is nothing more than an embarrassed act of self-defense. Yes, plants are alive, but one of the differences is the seeds and fruit of plants are created specifically to be eaten. In that way, the plant is able to spread and grow and create more food. If a plant's seeds and/or fruit are not eaten, it will be unable to propagate a wider area. In other words, plants benefit from being eaten. The same cannot be said for animals, which have a central nervous system necessary for the detection and avoidance of pain.

Veganism embraces instinct, which encompasses empathy, compassion and love, and, therefore, the elimination of suffering. Meat eaters, being sociopaths, will simply say and do anything, which is the antithesis of natural instinct, to alleviate their own perceived discomfort, and will deny any pain they bring to others.

Living in harmony and balance with nature is not only stress and guilt-free, but can even be a source of pleasure and comfort in itself. Instinct is a wonderful tool. Align yourself with it and you reap many and diverse benefits.

"Read nature; nature is a friend to truth."
– Edward Young

Going Against The Grain

One who swims with the current can move rapidly and effortlessly, and easily has enough energy left over to look up and see the sun shining. One who swims against the current must fight and struggle continuously, as to stop, even for a moment, could mean disaster. Once The Big Lie gets a grip on our psyches, it's hard to tell which way is up. For meat eaters there is a continual struggle to eat but to avoid thinking about it too deeply. Many of the gargantuan industries, such as meat and dairy, rely upon this denial for their riches.

> *"Awareness is bad for the meat business. Conscience is bad for the meat business. Sensitivity to life is bad for the meat business. DENIAL, however, the meat business finds indispensable."*
> *– Diet for a New America*, by John Robbins

Erecting a building on a poor foundation is a calamity waiting to happen, and a society not based upon a proper foundation of truth and love is just like that building, waiting to collapse. A society that revolves around meat is literally a disaster in progress. Eating meat not only causes disease and environmental hazards, but is in itself a brutal existence that encourages violence at every level. There are thousands of homicides in this country every year, yet no one knows why.

One day I happened to be watching CBS's *This Morning*. Harry Smith was talking to a government expert about the issue of crime. At the conclusion of the interview, Harry asked this expert what she felt was wrong with the soul of this country that allows this kind of activity. The expert answered, as all "experts" in this field do, by saying we need more money for various programs. Not only did she not answer the question, but she demonstrated some of the very problems with our "problem solvers." If the multitude of experts chattering around the world today are, in fact, experts, why do we still have all these problems? As hard as it may be to believe, crime, disease, pollution, inhumanity, etc., are not necessarily inherent in life, and using money to try to cure these ills does nothing but make them worse. To a great extent money is what created them in the first place.

Widespread chronic and degenerative disease, pollution, inhumanity, ecosystem breakdown, even street and domestic violence are simply the crumbling of a structure not built on a proper foundation. But these calamities, as you should now know from Chapter One, are not an unsolvable riddle. Getting to the root of problems is like learning mathematics – it only seems complicated when you don't understand it, but, once learned, it becomes an invaluable tool that makes problem solving elementary. Step back to the source.

The sad fact is that we have become a society whose truths are based upon its beliefs, rather than the other way around. It is this, The Big Lie, that abates our instinct and, as a result, we don't even know which way is up. Truth, as obscure as it may have become, remains truth and does not change in order to enhance careers, make money or accumulate power. Our experts, our problem solvers, are not looking so much to solve problems as they are looking to advance their careers, make money and accumulate power. Unfortunately, the solutions can never, and will never, be forthcoming using such a paradigm, which is the very antithesis of truth and instinct. The corruption of instinct that allows people to eat meat is the very same veil that paves the way for violence of every type.

"Civilization and violence are antithetical."
          – Dr. Martin Luther King Jr.

First Or Second Degree?

Some people argue that it is okay to kill animals as long as there isn't much pain inflicted. The very basis of this argument admits animals feel pain, but is an attempt to minimize the inhumanity of killing other living creatures. Does this argument mean that it is okay to kill as long as it is done without inflicting pain? Paradise can exist in a realm of murderous activity so long as there is no pain? If so, it should be perfectly acceptable to murder your family while they're sleeping. Your defense attorney would simply have to prove that the victims were not awake before they were shot to death.

"Your honor, my client has a cassette tape that was recorded the night of the murder, um, I mean the selfless act of humanity. Clearly, we can hear the alleged victim snoring loudly right up to the blast of the shotgun. I wish to enter into evidence Exhibit A, a photograph of the alleged crime scene, which clearly shows the shotgun blast cleanly and instantly removed the victim's head. I move to dismiss this case on the basis that my client is clearly not violent, as he went to great lengths, out of utter humanity, to make sure there was no pain inflicted."

Murder without pain is an interesting glimpse into the mind of "compassionate" meat eaters. To such people, The Big Lie is firmly entrenched in their minds, but it is garnished with a side order of sensitivity. This serves as a poignant case study in hypocrisy.

Sadly, many people teeter on the fence between The Big Lie and their innate empathy, so they eat "free range" animals raised on family farms because they don't want to be inhumane. This is simply denial, because exploiting, killing and eating animals, no matter how they are raised, is inhumane. Killing is a violation of another's individual sovereignty, a roadblock to paradise and an affront to God. If sensitivity is allowed to flourish, one can no longer exploit, kill and/or eat animals at all and, therefore, hypocrisy can be eliminated.

Truth and instinct tell us that the life of an animal is as important to it as your life is to you. Truth, instinct and veganism go hand in hand.

Meat On The Brain

The psychological impact of eating meat is severe. The very blunt bottom line is simply that one cannot feel completely connected to a world that one is playing a part to destroy. Depression and suicide are often byproducts of feelings of isolation. No matter how many smiling hamburgers are created by advertising agencies, we all know, at least subconsciously, the cows that died in order for us to eat them were not smiling. Our instincts cannot be completely denied, even if we bury them deep within our subconscious.

"Each man is haunted until his humanity awakens."
– William Blake

As a result of slick advertising and marketing, meat and animal products permeate almost every fiber of our existence, and, not coincidentally, so too now does Prozac®. Depression often accompanies sociopathy. It's actually a very natural extension, as sociopaths are only concerned with their own pain, disregarding others, so they wallow in the isolated self. To feel the pain of other people (or animals) and then to assist them in their need is the proper way out of sociopathy – and depression. Empathy and a connection to others is the natural antidote to the isolatedness of depression.

The psychological benefits of veganism are numerous. People who become vegan on ethical grounds experience a tremendous feeling of kinship and connectedness with the world, its inhabitants and its Creator. Vegans live in tune with their instincts; they don't have to hide from them. They certainly don't need drugs to hide from their own minds. Vegans can say they love animals and mean it, respecting and caring for their Creator's creations. Vegans know that they're not destroying the environment – our home of homes. A deep feeling of oneness, of kinship with the world, is a gift awarded to vegans, the value of which is not measurable by the gold standard. Paradoxically, some of the worst pain vegans can feel is not their own, but to see another in pain. Veganism is a club of humanity, and the best part is it's a club without membership restrictions. We can all share the wealth of humanity. The gates of paradise open widest when we all choose to join.

Get In The Know

Over the course of our lives we spend a great deal of time unconsciously struggling to return to our innate instinct and humanity, not knowing how to get there or even where "there" is. After all, every road leads us to a McDonald's with smiling hamburgers so adorable and cute that the world's problems couldn't possibly emanate from them, right? WRONG! Even the experts can't lead the way because almost all of them eat meat too and can't see past their own early indoctrination.

If you look for the truth hard enough you will find it, and veganism embraces these truths. Align, or more accurately realign, yourself with human instinct and finding truth becomes possible. It is my sincerest hope that this book will not only give you a road map back to your innate instinct, but supply the means and motivation to help you on your way. It's actually easier than you could possibly imagine, once you open your heart to the simple, yet beautiful, truths of nature. It is no coincidence that opening your heart to truths of nature is what instinct is all about.

Instinct, like love, should be recognized as far more than a feeling, object or drive, but rather as a skill and a behavior. Instinct allows us to recognize and embrace truth, which, in turn, strengthens and solidifies instinct, which then guides us through our lives recognizing more truths, which strengthens and solidifies instinct even more ...

Painful Rapture

Tuning in (or re-tuning in) to one's own instincts can be a painful experience, just as almost all detoxification programs are painful. As we step back, we begin to see how we lived our lives up to this point, and this can (and probably will) be difficult. As we begin to recognize truth, we begin to bear true responsibility for our lives and our behavior, and what we once saw as meat we now see as torture and murder. Be your own harshest critic.

> *"Think occasionally of the suffering of which you spare yourself the sight."* – Albert Schweitzer

Don't hide from this pain, but rather experience it and never forget it. Allow it to guide you into a new way of life – thoughtful, mindful, truthful, responsible, instinctual, humane and whole. Once through the pain, you will find yourself at peace with yourself and all existence. Be your own best friend.

> *"Vegetarian food leaves a deep impression on our nature. If the whole world adopts vegetarianism, it can change the destiny of humankind."* – Albert Einstein

Chapter 6

Human Physiology

The following chart will help demonstrate the physiological basis underlying the *fact* that human beings are, by nature, herbivores. It is a combination of several sources, including *The Comparative Anatomy of Eating*, by Milton R. Mills M.D. and *Vegan Nutrition: Pure and Simple*, by Michael Klaper M.D.

Physiological Comparisons

	Carnivores	Herbivores	Humans
Teeth: Incisors	Short and pointed	Broad, flattened and spade shaped	Broad, flattened and spade shaped
Teeth: Canines	Long, sharp and curved	Dull and short or long (for defense), or none	Short and blunted
Teeth: Molars	Sharp, jagged and blade shaped	Flattened with cusps	Flattened with nodular cusps
Facial Muscles	Reduced to allow wide mouth gape	Well-developed	Well-developed
Jaw Type	Angle not expanded	Expanded angle	Expanded angle
Jaw Joint Location	On same plane as molar teeth	Above the plane of the molars	Above the plane of the molars

	Carnivores	Herbivores	Humans
Jaw Motion	Shearing; minimal side-to-side motion	No shear; good side-to-side, front-to-back motion	No shear; good side-to-side, front-to-back motion
Major Jaw Muscles	Temporalis	Masseter and pterygoids	Masseter and pterygoids
Mouth Opening vs. Head Size	Large	Small	Small
Chewing	None; swallows food whole	Extensive chewing necessary	Extensive chewing necessary
Saliva	No digestive enzymes	Carbohydrate digesting enzymes	Carbohydrate digesting enzymes
Stomach Type	Simple	Simple or multiple chambers	Simple
Stomach Acidity	Less than or equal to pH 1 with food in stomach	pH 4 to 5 with food in stomach	pH 4 to 5 with food in stomach
Stomach Capacity	60 to 70% of total volume of digestive tract	Less than 30% of total volume of digestive tract	21 to 27% of total volume of digestive tract
Length of Small Intestine	3 to 6 times body length	10 to more than 12 times body length	10 to 11 times body length
Colon	Simple, short and smooth	Long, complex; may be sacculated	Long, sacculated
Liver	Can detoxify Vitamin A	Cannot detoxify Vitamin A	Cannot detoxify Vitamin A
Kidneys	Extremely concentrated urine	Moderately concentrated urine	Moderately concentrated urine
Nails	Sharp claws	Flattened nails or blunt hooves	Flattened nails
Pores	No pores; perspires through tongue	Perspires through pores	Perspires through pores

As you can plainly see, humans are herbivorous by design. We are the complete opposite of a carnivore. Some people may say that humans are omnivores, but the profile of a true omnivore is virtually identical to that of a carnivore. In fact, almost all carnivores are really omnivores. Herbivores eat no meat, yet nearly all carnivores eat some plants. Some people think humans have "fangs," which then qualifies them as carnivores. You simply need to look at the teeth of a true carnivore or omnivore, a lion for instance (or even a house cat), to understand what fangs really are. And, no, humans don't have them.

To be in tune with our natural, physical bodies, and thus to be healthy, means we must eat a plant-based diet. In fact, health is really just an extension of living naturally. Conversely, living in opposition to the natural self by eating meat and dairy will exact a huge toll on the human body, both directly and indirectly. If everyone put paint in their cars' gas tanks, not only would we have major problems with the cars themselves, but nobody would get to work on time, which would create other problems. Soon, the roads would become clogged with broken-down vehicles, and our favorite form of transportation would become the antithesis of movement. For humans, food is our fuel, and ingesting meat and dairy is like putting paint in our gas tanks. It is simply unfit for human consumption. Understanding even the basics of human physiology can be a powerful tool in gaining a true perspective on whether or not items should be categorized as food.

Meatiology

The meat and dairy industries aren't concerned with the truth of human physiology as much as they are with their bottom lines. In fact, the bottom line seems to be their only concern and, as a result, they will do just about anything to continue the lie. We've become accustomed to these lies from the meat and dairy industries because we've seen them time and time again on TV commercials, materials in school, etc. They are, however, merely propaganda campaigns generated to make money and to create an entire world of meat eaters who don't even question whether or not we should be eating meat and dairy in the first place. Each of us has the choice to hide behind the lie or stand up with the truth. Physiology is a truth of nature that can't be bought, sold, altered or spun into a glossy advertisement, and is as plain to see as the TV commercials that try to turn physiology into meatiology.

Watch And Learn

There are certain animals that we know to be herbivores and others that we know are carnivores. We can simply watch them eat what their instincts tell them to. (After all, animals in the wild don't have TV commercials telling them what to eat.) Some people say that humans are designed as carnivores but forget the fact that even the most successful carnivores don't eat meat three times a day. If they did, they'd be fat and sluggish (sound familiar?), in no condition to catch their next meal. Carnivores usually eat very sporadically, typically once a day at most, and sometimes once every several days. This allows them time to sleep, digest and excrete the putrefactive waste that eating meat produces. In fact, carnivores sleep or are inactive most of a twenty-four-hour day, while herbivores are awake and active for most of a twenty-four-hour day. Perhaps an appropriate slogan for the meat industry would be: "Sleep your life away: Eat meat and dairy."

Vegetable matter and flesh decompose very differently, and the digestion of these materials offers still more insight into recognizing which animals are carnivores and which are herbivores. Vegetable matter decomposes into basic chemical elements, whereas flesh actually rots as it decays. It is essential, therefore, that when flesh is eaten it pass through the body very quickly. Hence, a basic physiological trait of carnivores is that they have a very short intestine (about three times their body length) to facilitate this rapid passage of flesh. Conversely, a physiological similarity of herbivores is a very long intestine (ten to twelve times their body length), which is necessary for the absorption of vitamins, minerals and enzymes abundant in the plant foods they eat (or are supposed to eat, in the case of humans). A long intestine, such as in humans, gives rotting flesh too much time before it is excreted. This putrefactive flesh can then lead to many calamities, one of the more popular in meat-eating humans being colon cancer.

Nature's Rules

Align yourself with nature and you win; go against it and you lose. Look around, folks. We're losing big-time. Diseases such as heart disease, cancer and diabetes; environmental catastrophes such as deforestation, global warming, pollution of our drinking water supply, the breakdown of the ecosystem; and the lack of humanity in the world are all part and parcel of our meat-eating ways. (And we say we want paradise?) It needn't be this way. All we need to do is turn around and go with nature's current by becoming vegan. We'll all be so much better off, individually and collectively.

Scientists and researchers continue looking for cures for cancer and heart disease and for a solution to the obesity epidemic overwhelming the meat-eating world. However, until such time as we align ourselves with the truths of nature, this search will remain sheer folly. For every one step research moves society forward, somewhere, somehow, unnatural lifestyles take society two steps back.

Face Off

Some people claim to be die-hard realists and pragmatists, and concepts of truth and instinct have no place in their tangible world. These people can't be bothered with such intangible, abstract concepts (or what they consider to be intangible, abstract concepts). The physiology of the human body, however, offers such people direct and tangible evidence that we are herbivorous creatures. Sadly, most people who refuse to accept truths will often do so whether these truths are abstract, intangible or not, because in reality "abstract" and "intangible" are just words they use to avoid the real word for their philosophical position – denial.

We are all free to choose for ourselves to live in truth or hide behind lies. This choice is not only a gift, but a responsibility. Propaganda be damned. We must accept responsibility for our own lives and our own actions. Deciding to live by truth, to live in tune with our natural bodies, can seem scary, especially for people who have spent their entire lives eating meat and dairy (almost all of us). This is nothing more than a fear of the unknown, yet a whole new and beautiful world awaits those who penetrate this fear.

Living in tune with our natural physiology is the essence of peace and harmony, even for the physical body. As society makes this switch to veganism, peace and harmony will also prevail over the Earth. Peace and harmony, of any type, can never exist while we live in conflict with our natural physiology.

Chapter 7

Meat, Money & Power

*If a man's aspirations toward a righteous life are serious
... if he earnestly seeks a righteous life, his first act of
abstinence is from animal food, because, not to
mention the excitement of the passions produced by
such food, it is plainly immoral, as it requires an act
contrary to moral feeling, i.e. killing – and is called forth
only by greed."*

— Leo Tolstoy

The meat and animal product industries spend billions of
dollars on propaganda. If you're as old as me, think back to
when you were in school and you learned about the four food
groups, in which meat and dairy comprised a substantial
portion of the diet. Did you know that it was actually the
meat and dairy industries that paid for and furnished those
materials to the schools?

Now we have the food pyramid, which is an improvement over the four food groups, but not by much. The meat
and dairy industries weren't happy with it and fought
fervently against it, but lobbied heavily to at least get a
position on it. Obviously, the meat and dairy industries ply
their wares however they see fit, but we must recognize meat
and dairy for what they really are and exclude them entirely
from any list of food.

The Power Of The Pyramids

Throughout the millennia, people have believed that the pyramids of ancient Egypt hold great powers. Well, they're right. But before you get on an airplane to go bow before the great geometric hunks of stone, let me explain just what these phenomenal forces are.

Several thousand years ago there was a pharaoh, a king of sorts, with absolute power. In order for the king to sustain such power, he needed lieutenants, or seconds-in-command. Let's say the pharaoh had six of these. Now, in order for these lieutenants to be worthy of their rank, they each needed enforcers of their own. Let's say six each. This tier of thirty-six enforcers, in order to remain on that tier, needed some of their own pawns. And so it goes, all the way down until you get to the bottom, where most of the people reside. Such an arrangement has most of its room at the bottom. Such an arrangement is a pyramid, and it is how the entire world has been structured for thousands of years. Talk about phenomenal power!

The Egyptian pyramids were built as a symbol of the sovereign power of the pharaohs over all mankind. This is an evil structure because sovereignty belongs with every individual. Interestingly, the pharaohs did not build the pyramids themselves. It was actually the slaves who built them. The question that comes to mind is: Who could have actually had the most power?

> *"The biggest mistake you can make is to believe you work for someone else."*   – Unknown

The pyramids were built as a symbol of man's power over man. Even the very method of construction employed this philosophy. Consider a thousand men enslaved by one hundred men, who, in turn, report to an executive committee of ten men who get their orders from one man.

The pyramids are an evil caricature of the worst of mankind; a structure where each man steps on the others below him so that he may rise higher. This is a structure that has the least room at the top and the most room at the bottom. Sadly, it is more than a geometric shape. It is the structure of practically all present-day organizations and governments.

> *"I don't want to overthrow the government, I want to fire them."*   – Gallagher

The Egyptians built a testament to their serpentine empire based upon this philosophy, which, by its inherent structure, never allows for good, only control; a structure that pits man against man, where there are *no* winners; a structure to which we, unwittingly or otherwise, perpetually conform.

As time goes on, the pyramid grows. In our society, this is known as tenure or seniority. Those up above scoff at those below, but they need those down below to prop them up high. As long as we subscribe to this paradigm it will only get worse. Pyramids only grow at the bottom, and yet people don't like being at the bottom. Even those at the top pay the price in their stressful, never-ending escape from the grasp of those below. It's not the way the world is supposed to be. Nature is not sadistic.

Why do we conform to this ancient, evil form? The fact is we don't have to follow this misdirection. We can change this ill-fated cancer, but it'll take determination. Ask someone how hard it was to stop smoking after ten years of the habit. But it was for the best, right? Well, this is a five-thousand-year habit. Expect some withdrawal pangs, but focus on what lies ahead.

If the way of the pyramid is bad, which it is, then perhaps the exact opposite way is good. Invert the pyramid (figuratively speaking only, otherwise you could get a hernia!). This puts the most room at the top and actually inhibits being at the bottom. In real terms, inverting the pyramid means being an individual. It means laying to rest our warped notions of authority that serve no one, not even those in authority. It means struggling with the realization and responsibility that you have the ultimate power over you. So, take control over your own life, or don't complain when somebody does it for you. But be sure to temper that with the fact that you only have power over you. If you give away your control, don't be mad at someone who takes it or at how they use it once they have it. You can, however, seek solace in the knowledge that you can almost always get it back. Just take it. I know this is a tough concept for most to accept considering society's indoctrination, but remember exactly who it was who actually built the pyramids.

Remove yourself from the pyramid. Don't prop anybody else up, nor require anybody to prop you up.

"Don't walk in front of me, I may not follow. Don't walk behind me, I may not lead. Just walk beside me and be my friend." – Albert Camus

The next time somebody says, "Vote for me and, as your leader, *I will serve you*," before casting your ballot, please call me. I have several bridges I need to sell. But seriously, rather than casting your ballot for someone to "lead you," cast your "ballot" for yourself, if you will, and live according to the highest order of humanity – individual sovereignty.

Individual sovereignty is a form of self-rule. In the realm of individual sovereignty, every individual is entitled to life, liberty and the pursuit of happiness to the fullest extent, so long as they don't infringe on any other individual's right to the same. Individual sovereignty is not a license to violate others, but rather a huge responsibility to care for the self and allow others to do the same. An extension of individual sovereignty would be to actually help others help themselves. Individual sovereignty comes from proper love. Love all to the fullest extent and that allows all to pursue individual sovereignty. Without individual sovereignty society will remain largely uncivilized and inhumane, no matter which "leaders," or how many of them, hold office.

> *"Liberty means responsibility. That is why most men dread it."*   – George Bernard Shaw

Every government embraces and pursues sovereignty of nations, but they outright scorn the notion of individual sovereignty, as they know that would be the end of government as we know it. More interesting is that even in the complete absence of leaders, society will reach its potential when (and not until) it comes to respect and embrace the sovereignty of the individual above all else. This will be best for each of us, individually and collectively. In fact, respecting the sovereignty of the individual is an intrinsic component of veganism, as it is dishonorable to violate any other beings' rights to their sovereignty. Within the practical application of a vegan way of life, getting on top of the pyramid is not nearly as important as becoming part of humanity. In truth, getting on top is the antithesis of creating kinship with the world. Eating another's flesh instantly dissolves kinship with the world.

Veganism is the fundamental tool for removing the ancient and evil power of the pyramids, and allowing all of us, God's family, to make our journey on the road to paradise. Allowing others to make their journey helps us to make ours. The complete actualization of paradise requires us all to journey together. Everyone who lives and breathes upon this planet must have complete right to life, liberty and the pursuit of happiness to the fullest extent, while not infringing on any other's right to the same. Veganism (even the letter "V") is the inverse of the pyramids.

The Spanish Connection

When sovereignty of the individual is replaced by a belief in a hierarchy, just about any means can be justified for getting on top. Money is the most common and time-tested excuse used toward this end. In fact, money was created by those who needed a portable device for trading their wealth.

I remember learning in school about Christopher Columbus, and I was inspired by how he courageously set sail for the New World, and how Spain financed this noble endeavor. What our teachers forgot to tell us (or never knew themselves) was *why* Christopher Columbus had an interest in setting sail at all, and especially why Spain financed this project.

Beef (murdered cows) had become the backbone of the Spanish government's wealth. As the beef trade (and their pyramid) grew, the value of this commodity soared. The problem was that there was still no really good way of preserving the carcasses. A government is not a government without its money or control (one and the same), and rotting carcasses were ruining Spain's gig.

Spain had no interest in serving humanity, though Queen Isabella did appear to like the idea of spreading the word to any "heathen" natives Columbus came across. Spain's primary interest was in protecting its wealth, growing the pyramid and ridding the land of the foul smell emanating from all its cattle cadavers. Columbus stepped in and offered to find Spice Island, seeking to return with a bounty of spices to preserve the carcasses and conceal the odors, and expand Spain's business interests. Spain funded this venture because its very survival, its economy, revolved around the flesh and blood of murdered docile cattle. The more efficiently Spain could market its product, the more money it would have and, consequently, the more power it would have; power not to serve the Earth, but to own it. However, man cannot and will not own the Earth. The Earth owns man. Any attempt to alter this simple truth will always lead to catastrophe eventually.

By the way, it was Spain that introduced cattle to the New World.

Lessons In Insight

You've probably heard the saying "The more things change, the more they stay the same." I was never fully sure what that meant until I attended the National Food Policy Conference in Washington, D.C. The purpose of the conference is to assemble people with an interest in the food industry, both public and private, in order to address any current issues and make our food supply safer, healthier, more abundant and less expensive. Sounds pretty good, right?

Insight Builder #1 – One of the very first speakers was Philip Fletcher, then CEO of ConAgra. ConAgra is one of the nation's largest slaughterhouses. No matter how well concealed, by distance or walls, the fact is ConAgra murders millions upon millions of innocent, sentient animals, the flesh of which can never, ever be made safe for human consumption because nature never, ever intended it to go into a human stomach.

Insight Builder #2 – Ellen Haas, then the under secretary for Food, Nutrition and Consumer Services for the United States Department of Agriculture, also spoke at the conference. In her address, "Who's Watching Out For The Kids?", she discussed her brand new $20 million project that was to be known as "Team Nutrition." Team Nutrition was a program aimed at getting kids to eat better. Team Nutrition was _heavily_ supported by the beef and dairy industries. The more things change, the more they stay the same.

The Revolving Door

Many government officials, including those in the Food and Drug Administration (FDA) and the United States

Department of Agriculture (USDA), leave office to take lucrative positions in the private sector, including food and drug businesses. They do this for short periods and then go back to work for the government again, such as with the FDA and the USDA, and write and enforce government policy that is supposed to be overseeing the very industries that have just enriched them. In a relatively short period of time, these people can go back and forth from the public to the private sector many times, writing favorable public policy and being rewarded for it by large corporations and industries. This "revolving door," as it is referred to in Washington, D.C., offers a glimpse into exactly who is trying to create a "healthy, safe and abundant food supply" for us. These people strive to keep the pyramids growing. That is why it is imperative that we make our food choices our own responsibility. If we don't, someone else who has little interest in our well-being will do it for us.

"Each act of denial, conscious or unconscious, is an abdication of our power to respond."
– Joanna Rogers Macy

Money In The Bank

The United States government heavily subsidizes the meat and dairy industries, so much so that if the subsidies were removed meat prices would be many times what they are now. Conversely, fruit, vegetable and grain producers are forced to destroy crops in order to keep prices high. This artificial price manipulation is why vegetable products appear to be expensive today compared to meat. Though it may be hard to believe, plant-based foods, such as fruits, vegetables, grains, nuts, seeds and legumes could, and should, be practically free. In VeganWorld, plant foods would be so plentiful they would be available for the taking.

Imagine if you sat down to a light meal of some tomatoes and cucumbers. Each single fruit has many seeds. If you were to take a few and plant them in the ground, tomatoes and cucumbers would, henceforth, be free. The same goes for apples, pineapples, peas, peanuts and every other fruit, vegetable, grain, legume and nut you can imagine. The more food that is grown and eaten, the more food there could actually be. This is in stark contrast to meat, which has a diminishing-return effect, creating an ever-decreasing supply of food.

Because meat has become the centerpiece of our diet, it's hard to believe that it is the underlying culprit of many of the Earth's ills. A great many dollars are riding on your not knowing this.

Meat Is The Seed Of All Evil

"For the love of money is the root of all evil."
– 1 Timothy 6:10

What Timothy may have forgotten to say is that meat is the seed of all money. It was largely when man first attempted to claim ownership over animals that there needed to be some sort of device of ownership and tool for trading what was now owned – the animal's flesh. Money enabled man to first control livestock and, subsequently, other men. Without the pursuit of money it would be difficult, if not impossible, to control others. Without controlling others, there would be no slaves. Without controlling others, there would be no meat. Ownership and control replaces freedom and individual sovereignty. But individual sovereignty is what a good society must be based upon. Any society based on ownership and control will also always be violent (to gain the ownership and control). Therefore, it is not necessarily only the violence that makes society evil, but the control.

Sometimes violence is just a byproduct of someone attempting to control others and those others attempting to defend themselves.

> *"As long as there are slaughterhouses, there will be battlefields."*
>   – Leo Tolstoy

The Freedom Fighters

Freedom is a magnificent gift. We should honor those who help the cause of freedom, and we should never waiver in our resolve for freedom … freedom for all, that is. You are either a freedom fighter or you're not.

In 1990, Operation Desert Shield, and the subsequent Operation Desert Storm, seemed to solidify the "free world's" resolve for freedom, at least in a political sense. There was, quite literally, a run on U.S. flags. People sat back and watched live on television as the allied air forces – you know, the good guys – beat up on the evil empire of Saddam Hussein.

Before complete and total euphoria took over, the war was winding down. At least *our* war was winding down. Saddam Hussein then vented his frustration at his defeat by launching a most vicious attack on the Kurds in the north of Iraq. A massacre was unfolding and the "freedom fighters" were nowhere to be seen.

> *"I love my country but I fear my government."*
>   – Unknown

It may be true that we occasionally fight for freedom, but unfortunately we fight far more frequently to grow our pyramids for our own agendas. Those agendas are always about money, and money is often about controlling others – people and animals. But freedom, in truth, is a divine and unalienable right for all who live upon Planet Earth. Anyone who endeavors to take away another's freedom is committing the filthiest of crimes.

> *"If a man wants freedom why keep birds and animals in cages?"*
> – Leonardo da Vinci

The United States of America was built upon some magnificent principles: "… that all men are created equal … with certain unalienable rights … life, liberty, and the pursuit of happiness;" and "… justice for all" are two that immediately come to mind. In fact, the Declaration of Independence states that "We hold these truths to be self-evident." But these are only philosophies which, like emotions, mean nothing without the proper behavior to back them up. If these are truths, self-evident at that, shouldn't they be categorical? Was the Kurds' right to freedom not self-evident?

In America today most people spend their lives in pursuit of money and power, believing this is the source of happiness. But getting to the top, controlling others, even eating other living things does nothing to help you achieve happiness. There are 168 hours in a week. If we sleep eight hours a night, work twelve hours a day (including getting ready and traveling to work) for five days a week, this leaves a grand total of fifty-two hours for everything else in our life – family, hobbies, etc. This means less than thirty-one percent of our lives is about life's enjoyment and fulfillment. If we factor in the time it takes to shop for food and clothes and to do other chores, the percentage gets even bleaker. How much time does this leave us to serve others? After all, serving others is proper love, and it is the very meaning of life. We are spending our lives chasing after everything but that which we ought to be pursuing the most vigorously.

"I am absolutely convinced that no wealth in the world can help humanity forward, even in the hands of the most devoted worker in this cause. The example of great and pure individuals is the only thing that can lead us to noble thoughts and deeds. Money only appeals to selfishness and irresistibly invites abuse. Can anyone imagine Moses, Jesus, or Gandhi armed with the money-bags of Carnegie?" – Albert Einstein

We are a society that pursues monetary riches above all else. This creates rich people who, in turn, create poor people. Yes, rich people need poor people. If we were all rich, who would clean the mansions? There is nothing necessarily wrong with pursuing comforts, but at what cost? If we pursue external riches at the expense of internal riches, i.e. wisdom, contentment and happiness, we may be far poorer than our padded bank accounts suggest. We have become a society that celebrates and embraces monetary riches, yet just try to find a sage. All the while, we are spinning out of control just trying to get to work on time. Then our paychecks help to fuel the backward economy of meat.

The old saying is true: money can't buy happiness. Happiness comes from love. It is kinship with one's world and all its inhabitants that offers true peace and contentment, and this is the exclusive blueprint of love. Kinship with the world is the only way to happiness, and it is, therefore, the highest order of wealth. To the greatest extent, we live our lives in stark contrast to those old, wise sayings.

Unfortunately, while there are those who wish to control others, wars for freedom may sometimes be necessary. Very few wars, however, have been fought for that reason. Most wars are, in truth, about a reallocation of power and wealth. Freedom and sovereignty of the individual is the highest form, actually the only form, of a true civilization. In just the same way that the thorn stands ready and vigilant, yet unobtrusive, to protect the rose, we must stand ready and vigilant, yet unobtrusive, to protect peace and freedom. We should do this not for our own nearsighted aggrandizement and pyramid growth, but simply and purely to protect what is just. This is the essence of human and humane responsibility. In order to put this philosophy into practice, all mankind will have to be vegan. From this standpoint, wars to help all people and all animals (yes, even cows) achieve freedom may be necessary. You are either a freedom fighter or you're not. Most freedom being denied in our world today can be corrected without machine guns, by simply removing flesh from our dinner plates.

Rally 'Round The Flag, Boys

The President of the United States would never go on television and announce that we are going to war because his political party thinks it would help him win reelection in the face of domestic policies that may be failing dismally. Rather, he will go on television and announce that "freedom hangs in the balance" and "we must secure freedom for our children." Such an announcement plays on people's emotions and we do the "patriotic" thing; we rally 'round the flag. But so do the people of the county that is soon to be our enemy. In fact, the leaders of all countries tell their people whatever it takes to incite them against their friends from distant lands, or soon-to-be opponents. If it is the patriotic and right thing to support our president in his call to war, even if the reasons seem somewhat spurious, how can we fault our "enemies" for doing the same? Just like us, they have been led to believe that we stand in the way of their happiness. But don't expect the leaders, ours or theirs, to let you see it that way.

"Universal responsibility is feeling for other people's suffering just as we feel for our own. It is the realization that even our enemy is entirely motivated by the quest for happiness. We must recognize that all human beings want the same thing we want."
                                    – The XIV Dalai Lama

Should we fight for freedom? Unequivocally, yes. After all, we are either freedom fighters or we're not. But first we need to recognize and then correct how *we* are denying others their freedom – even if it is on our dinner plates. Be grateful for the freedom you have and allow others the same.

Rallying around the flag can be a very dangerous activity. Just in recent times alone the Nazis did it, the Japanese did it, the Iranians and Iraqis did it, and it is has been no less inappropriate and dangerous here in America. To support a piece of land solely because an accident of birth means you happen to have been born there is absurd. In fact, the very notion of individual countries is absurd. Most modern-day nations were artificially created by violent people seeking wealth and power, and the borders are constantly changing as one side or the other fights its way to grab another few acres.

Immigration is a hotly debated topic these days. If nations fight to protect borders around their turf, how can they scorn the Bloods and Crips for doing the same? There are no borders in nature. There are no enemies in truth, only fellow human beings.

One of the greatest enablers of war, and a true enemy of humanity, is patriotism. If you want to be patriotic or loyal to something, be loyal to principles that you believe are just, not to a piece of land, a president or a flag. It is essential that we embrace the fundamental and behavioral aspects of what we are all really fighting for – love and happiness – and the freedom of all to pursue it. Love respects the sovereignty of each and every individual, and means treating all others the way we would like all others to treat us.

It is disturbing to consider that hundreds of millions of people will rally around the flag over, say, oil interests and consider this a noble fight, a fight by the "freedom fighters." Yet most of these same people think nothing of the ten billion sentient animals that are imprisoned, brutalized and murdered every single year. Then, if a few animal rights "activists" try to stop the brutality and enslavement, they are looked upon as weirdos or extremists. Many in government, who would consider themselves to be freedom fighters, count animal rights activists as terrorists.

Leo Tolstoy examined the absurdity of a society that looks upon an individual killing another individual as murder, yet embraces as a good and noble deed when many individuals get together to do some killing and call it "war." It is an even greater absurdity that society scorns those who categorically refuse to engage in the murder of any living thing.

> *"When a man has pity on all living creatures then only is he noble."*
>   – The Buddha

Albert Schweitzer wrote of our age as being "filled with contempt for thought." He also wrote in his autobiography, *Out of My Life and Thought*, that "… organized political, social, and religious associations of our time are at work convincing the individual not to develop convictions through his own thinking but to assimilate the ideas they present to him."

People who think are a threat to the pyramidal philosophy and, therefore, to corporate bodies, churches and governments. Consequently, schools sponsored by churches or governments don't teach people to think, but rather to conform and to perpetuate the nonsense. Those pyramidal entities actually strive ardently to discredit individual thought.

The true goal of war, as well as the art of war, is not to annihilate the enemy but to win them over. Over two thousand years ago, in *The Art of War*, Sun Tzu, an ancient Chinese philosopher and military strategist, wrote, "Supreme excellence consists in breaking the enemy's resistance without fighting." To seek to destroy someone for destruction's sake is evil.

Those who live by oppressing, controlling, brutalizing and even killing others, and refuse to yield to humanity, must be stopped. This is not a political statement, but a categorical necessity of truth and humanity, and therefore must apply to each and every one of us in our behavior toward *all* others. It is a responsibility. For a freedom fighter to truly be a freedom fighter, he or she must fight to prevent one person or group of people having power over another. Freedom fighters must help those who can't help themselves. Moreover, each one of us is either a freedom fighter or not in our everyday behavior.

"As long as men massacre animals, they will kill each other. Indeed, he who sows the seeds of murder and pain cannot reap joy and love."   – Pythagoras

Chapter 8

Violence

"The world is a comedy to those that think; a tragedy to those that feel." — Horace Walpole

The magnitude of violence in our society is alarming. Street violence is at nightmarish levels, and domestic violence is terrifyingly common. Our "experts" continually resort to increasing budgets for various programs, as though that's going to cure the problem. All bigger budgets accomplish is keeping the experts employed, putting bigger and bigger band-aids over bigger and bigger problems.

A meat-eating society requires massive killing and is, therefore, massively violent. Plus, the very ability that makes eating animals possible, denial of another's rights and sovereignty, is the very ability that creates much of the world's violence. In truth, almost all violence emanates from the top of society, not the bottom.

"While we ourselves are the living graves of murdered beasts, how can we expect any ideal conditions on this Earth?" — George Bernard Shaw

Eating meat is violence. Everyone who eats meat is contributing to the violence three times a day. A myriad of sociologists, psychologists and other experts spend countless hours and millions of dollars trying to find an answer to all this violence. Why haven't they? Because the answers cannot be forthcoming when even the experts engage in and, therefore, overlook the very practice that creates much of the violence.

"The dad who comes home and kicks the dog is probably just warming up."
– Washington Humane Society

It is a known fact that virtually all violent people abused animals at some point in their lives. Animal abuse, as any sociologist, psychologist or behaviorist can tell you, is an integral part of the personality profiles of criminally violent people. The act of kicking a dog is considered animal abuse. But what about killing an animal and eating its dead body? Is this not the most extreme form of abuse? Whether sociologists want to categorize eating animals as abuse or not, the truth remains that over ten billion animals are murdered every year. As a result, nearly 300 million Americans are abusive toward animals and, consequently, are massively violent. That our street thugs are violent is no mystery at all in a society that not only turns a blind eye to violence but actually applauds it – and eats it.

Moreover, it is silly to know that a vegan diet is good for the body yet completely disregard its benefit for the mind and soul.

"Out of 135 criminals, including robbers and rapists, 118 admitted that when they were children they burned, hanged and stabbed domestic animals."
– Ogonyok (Russian weekly magazine)

No matter how many layers of The Big Lie cover it up, butchery permeates all aspects of society. Traditionally, we've looked at violent criminals as evil thugs, overlooking the fact that we created these evil thugs. For a host of sordid reasons, a meat-eating society is the breeding ground for *all* violence. Only as each person stops his involvement in the butchery will society benefit accordingly.

Desensitize, Desensitize!

Like it or not, eating animals is contributing not only to the actual violence that plagues our world, but to the desensitization that makes violence possible in the first place. A meat-eating society, which is necessarily compulsive and sociopathic, lives by desensitization and justification. If mankind truly behaved as humanely as we like to think we do, there would be no possible way we could kill and eat one breathing, feeling animal, much less ten billion a year.

Most people would run to a dog's rescue if they saw it being kicked, yet many of them would go home afterward and eat a chicken salad or a hot dog or a tuna sandwich and think nothing of it. Now, I don't know about you, but I'd rather be kicked than eaten. The ability to eat a hot dog or tuna sandwich comes, in part, from desensitization. It is essential to desensitize oneself to any empathy toward the animals in order to be able to eat them. This desensitization, which is so essential to a meat-eating society, is the very seed of all violence.

Some people may think it silly to equate people such as Charles Manson or Jeffrey Dahmer to meat eaters. Some branches in a tree simply grow higher than others. But make no mistake about from where the seeds come. If Charles Manson was taught as a young child to respect all life (the essential meaning of veganism), could he possibly have participated in brutally killing people? If Jeffrey Dahmer's innate empathy had been allowed to flourish instead of being suppressed, could he have killed and eaten his victims?

Even those of us who aren't considered to be violent, yet eat meat, are full-time employees of the violence factory.

Education?

"My refusing to eat flesh occasioned an inconveniency, and I was frequently chided for my singularity, but, with this lighter repast, I made the greater progress, for greater clearness of head and quicker comprehension."
– Benjamin Franklin

Children go to school to learn, and all too often what children learn is how to kill. What's worse, these children learn it is perfectly alright to kill. This "education" teaches children that brutality is okay if you are bigger and stronger than your victim, especially if your victim can't speak out.

One widely taught practice in our schools is dissection. It initially breaks the hearts of many teenagers to engage in this drill. It then hardens them against their innate empathy and humanity. Peer pressure and the fear of speaking up reinforces this evil process. Who is there to speak up for the child, the principles of humanity or God's weakest of sentient creatures?

"To my mind, the life of a lamb is no less precious than the life of a human being. I should be unwilling to take the life of a lamb for the sake of the human body. I hold that, the more helpless the creature, the more entitled it is to protection by man from the cruelty of man."
– Mahatma Gandhi

In the case of dissection, the teachers explain that it's okay to kill the frog or the mouse because these are "animals." (I suppose this is in contrast to humans, which, I guess, are minerals, uh, I mean vegetables.) From this early indoctrination, people live their entire lives certain of such hypocritical nonsense. It is this very desensitization and confusion that paves the way for violence of every kind and magnitude.

> *"Teaching a child not to step on a caterpillar is as valuable to the child as it is to the caterpillar."*
> – Bradley Miller

The curriculum in practically all high school biology classes includes dissection of small animals. Why? What do children really learn from this that they can't learn from a picture, a plastic rendering or a computer model? In fact, many children are so frazzled by the sight of the dead and mutilated animal they can't retain anything on that day other than remembering the horrid and adrenaline-producing sight. In addition, the lesson of dissection they take with them on their life's journey has nothing whatsoever to do with biology, but rather is a lesson in sociopathy and desensitization of their innate empathy and humanity. The parents, the teachers, the entire educational system and society as a whole sanction the lesson that it's okay to kill a little animal. In truth, anyone who sanctions and/or teaches that killing is okay is in dire need of a real education themselves. Participating in any process that includes a murdered animal is murder by way of complicity and is further destruction of paradise.

Any accountant can tell you, what goes on one side of a ledger must also go on the other side. This is the essence of a balance sheet. Likewise, one cannot kill an animal (for food, clothing, entertainment or otherwise) and then effectively teach a child that violence and killing are wrong. It just will not balance out. Such an attempt, however, will teach children three things. Firstly, it desensitizes them to empathy. Secondly, it teaches children how to be violent. Thirdly, it teaches them how to be hypocrites to such an extent they can't even see it themselves, perfect conditioning for a lifelong commitment to The Big Lie. By the time most of us graduate high school, we have strong sociopathic foundations. And paradise becomes an abstract concept.

Higher Learning

At lunchtime and in science classes our education system teaches that killing is perfectly okay. So why don't we understand the proliferation of violence in our society? While some situations and some violence may seem more barbaric than others, it is just that some branches grow higher than others. All come from the very same seeds. From the proper perspective, it's not that difficult to understand. It may, however, be difficult to accept, but this is a natural part of the transformation away from eating meat. In fact, all of us who have made the journey must first come to the painful realization of the enormous pain we've inflicted on others. It is actually at this point of realization, and the refusal to deny the truth any longer, that we can learn the most important lessons.

We must teach children that all killing is wrong and that all life is sacred. But again, unfortunately, this lesson is impossible to impart to children while we live in contrast to this most basic principle of humanity. As a result, we must make humanity our individual responsibility, which, in practical terms, means giving up meat and animal products, for openers.

Rebels Without A Cause

Many children are rebellious and more and more children are criminally violent. Again, nobody understands why. Rebellion often stems from violated instincts. Try to stop someone from breathing and see if he rebels. Rebellion itself is often an act of instinct when something is amiss. In children, rebellion is a mutational reaction, an inability to correctly respond to a given set of circumstances. All human beings are innately loving and caring until such time as they are taught otherwise, and then rebellion and violence are sure to follow.

Whether parents actively abuse their children or simply offer them a piece of an animal to eat (an animal that the children instinctively love), the children's instincts naturally begin the defense mechanism of rebellion. Young children cannot consciously understand what they are rebelling against (especially in the case of eating animals), but their instincts and their innate empathy and humanity know something is very wrong.

> **Child:** "Mommy, did these chicken nuggets come from that same cute chicken I saw playing in the field yesterday?"
> **Mother:** "Oh, no, sweetheart. Of course not."
> **Child:** "Okay, Mommy."

By the time children are in their teens, they are already so lost in confusion, they simply rebel. Unfortunately, they have already been so conditioned by The Big Lie, they don't even know what they are rebelling against. Neither do their parents, nor the "experts." They are rebelling because they haven't been allowed to grow the way nature intended – loving, caring and empathetic. Millions of young children insist they love animals while eating a Big Mac. After a few years, many of these same children will become the enigmatic rebels and nobody will understand their raw emotions.

Lessons From The Wild Child

Though most reported cases of "feral children" are folklore, there are actually a few rare documented cases of children who became completely isolated from human society. These children often seem mentally impaired and exhibit considerable difficulty learning to walk upright, are almost incapable of learning a human language and display no interest in the human activity around them.

Clearly, our earliest conditioning virtually mandates how we will live our lives. Sociopathic upbringing makes it near impossible to fully understand empathy, love, truth, compassion, etc. Many vegans don't understand why, with an insurmountable stack of data to support veganism as the way we all should live, most still insist on flesh. It isn't that hard to understand when we consider the insights gathered from feral children. Brain scans of feral children show an actual loss of development.

Many enlightened vegans weren't always vegan. In some ways this is promising news because this means there is a process of "detoxification" that we can use to attain an enlightened plateau of living where empathy, love, truth, compassion, etc., do prevail. This is a choice you must bring to the forefront of your consciousness and then make an enlightened decision. The stepping back method is instrumental in this process.

The bad news is that we are still creating enormous dysfunction in our children. It is preposterous to believe that we can raise children to be decent and loving human beings by teaching them that killing is perfectly okay. It must stop, but it must first stop with you.

Meat's Impact On Emotion, Aggression And Violence

"Besides agreeing with your aims for aesthetic and moral reasons, it is my view that a vegetarian manner of living by its purely physical effect on the human temperament would most beneficially influence the lot of mankind."
— Albert Einstein

People who swallow vitamin C have vitamin C in their bodies. It's a silly thing to have to point out because it simply goes without saying. It should be equally silly, but unfortunately is not, to point out that people who swallow fear, violence and aggression have these elements in their bodies.

Think about a time when you were frightened and how your body responded to that fear. Many hormones are released to help you in the fight or flight response that can take you out of danger. Likewise, there are many types of hormones in the bloodstream and the flesh of an animal being killed, such as adrenaline and epinephrine, that are released to assist their natural defenses and their will to live. By eating animal parts containing these hormones, which is unavoidable when eating a murdered animal, you are ingesting fear and aggression. Eating fish, most of which suffocate when taken out of the water, not to mention the pain of the hooks and nets, can offer up a host of aggression hormones. Further, it's silly to think that your offspring's DNA won't be adversely affected by all the fear and aggression hormones you've ingested. It's no more complex, albeit far more uncomfortable, than the vitamin C example. A violent society creating future ever-increasingly violent societies.

Through all my research I have not been able to locate even one rapist or murderer in prison who is vegan or vegetarian. In response to this observation, some people like to point out that Hitler was a vegetarian in a moronic attempt to disparage the philosophy. But, as I said, it is moronic. The fact is, because of his poor health, Hitler's doctors suggested that he become vegetarian, but he refused. Some of his favorite foods were, in fact, various flesh products. Even if Hitler had decided to follow his doctor's advice, he would have been doing so out of selfish reasons – his health. While such a rarity as a violent vegan may exist somewhere, the big picture offers tremendous insight into aggressive and violent personalities and from where they may be getting their aggression and violence. There is no question that aggression and violence are an integral part of a meat-eating world, whereas vegans, be it due to philosophy or chemically (makes no difference), are almost exclusively gentle, kind and respectful of life.

Why Do Bad Things Happen To Good People?

Disease and violence plague mankind, and when somebody says, "Why do bad things happen to good people?" I can't help but ask, "What good people?" The human race is, by far, the most savage and violent killing machine the Earth has ever known. Only when we become the caring, empathetic, humane stewards of the land that God and nature intended us to be do we deserve to ask such a question. Ironically, when we do finally realize our humane potential, we will no longer need to ask such superfluous questions.

After the horrible events of September 11, 2001, many people asked, "Where was God on 9/11?" As someone who abhors murder of all kind, I can't help but think of the BILLIONS of animals that would like to ask, "Where was God on 9/9, 9/10, 9/11, 9/12, 9/13, 9/14 . . . ?"

Society's eating animals is a mutiny against God.

The Paradise Zone

Ask someone to close his or her eyes for a few moments and picture paradise. Once your subject has visualized this image, ask him or her to describe it. Almost always, the description includes "peace and harmony for all." We usually hear a lot about peace on Earth and harmony for all around the holidays, when everybody is busy cooking up a Christmas ham or turkey, or a brisket of beef for Hanukkah. So, peace on Earth for whom, exactly? Certainly not for the cow or the pig or the turkey and, with equal certitude, since all things are connected, not for man.

So now, for a moment, close your eyes and picture paradise. This time, picture paradise at 7:30 a.m. on Wednesday morning. All of us have arisen after a beautiful night's sleep – after all, this is paradise. The breakfast bell chimes throughout our utopian land. On this particular morning, however, Johnny feels like some nice crisp bacon. If you allow your innate empathy to paint this picture, you would put yourself in the bacon's place, or, more accurately, the pig's place. (The word "bacon" is just a nice way of denying what we are eating.) Now you are a docile, harmless animal with keen senses. You enjoy nothing more than rummaging about the land happily, living your life in sync with your initial portrait of paradise. But, this morning, Johnny wants to eat you. At that instant, every horror movie that could ever possibly be made materializes into vivid reality; scenes at which Stephen King himself would marvel. Someone is now coming after you to kill you and eat your flesh.

First the chase, long and grueling. In utter fear, you rush out of your home. Disbelief and confusion vainly attempt to guide your every step – an experience similar to nightmares in which you try to run or scream but can't; only this is reality. You squeal for help, but those who can help don't understand your screams. Besides, at this point, many of them wouldn't mind a piece of your ass either, so they get in on the chase. (On a side note, this description isn't nearly as horrific as reality. At least in this story, it is inferred that the pig had some portion of his life to live as nature intended. Most pigs are nothing more than products of factory farms, where they are kept chained up in cages. They have no way of even attempting to run. Many pigs raised in factory farms can hardly even stand.)

The horrific ante is upped with the capture, which in itself is painful and agonizing. Shortly you'll be food and, as a result, your comfort and well-being is hardly a consideration.

You are no longer your mother's child. From this point forward you are worth about two dollars a pound.

The coffee's on and you're led to the slaughter. Frightened, tired, hungry, thirsty and confused, you put up one last fight, but your once energetic and happy body is no match for the steel shackles. You're hoisted upside down by your feet, the pain so intense you can't even scream anymore. One joint is dislocated and a couple of vertebrae crack from the force of the violent machine. You hang there for a few agonizing moments and then . . .

I will spare you the final horrors of the slaughterhouse, but this scenario is just the smallest tip of the largest iceberg. But now try to visualize paradise. You can't? Of course not. It's gone. The seeds of violence, crime, greed, pollution and disease have been bountifully sown. Peace on Earth is now but a greeting card slogan and, along with "Thou shalt not kill," becomes a selectively used slogan for selfish and greedy purposes.

Contrary to popular opinion, one cannot profit from another's demise. We must face up to the genocide of the millennium and turn to a vegan diet. Not just because it's healthy, which it is. Not just because it's economically prudent, which it is. Not just because it's environmentally friendly and sustainable, which it is. We must turn to a plant-based diet because we are human, because we are humane. In much the same way that a typical Saturday night babysitter who has been granted temporary dominion over your child has the choice to care for it or to molest it, we have a choice to care for each other and the world or to destroy it. Just as we'd hope the babysitter would apply her dominionship responsibly and with love for our children, we should also behave in like kind with our underlings. It is this very choice that determines good or evil behavior. We must own up to the responsibility to care for our world and its inhabitants. To be human means to protect *all* those who can't protect themselves, whereas "might over right" is undeniably the meat eaters' manifesto. Only when we choose a kind, humane way of eating – a vegan diet – can we create and sustain the kind of world we all claim we want. It deeply saddens me to report that in a meat-eating society there are no sweet little old ladies. Only when we choose a vegan diet based on humanity can we consider ourselves worthy of being labeled human beings. Then, and only then, will we have sweet little old ladies, kind gentlemen and, yes, caring, playful, nonviolent children.

> *"Until he extends his circle of compassion to all living things, man will not himself find peace."*
> – Albert Schweitzer

Well, I really must run. I have to get some shark cartilage to keep myself from getting cancer. Never mind the fact that when all the sharks are gone (and they're vanishing rapidly) cancer will pale in comparison to the disasters that will face us. If you believe that health can exist in a society that kills, consider this: What if eating a human heart gave us eternal life? What type of world would it be? Who would, in fact, have eternal life? More to the point, who would want eternal life in such a world?

> *"My situation is a solemn one: Life is offered to me on condition of eating beef-steaks. But death is better than cannibalism. My will contains directions for my funeral, which will be followed not by mourning coaches, but by oxen, sheep, flocks of poultry, and a small traveling aquarium of live fish, all wearing white scarves in honor of the man who perished rather than eat his 'fellow creatures.' It will be, with the exception of Noah's Ark, the most remarkable thing of the kind ever seen."*
> – George Bernard Shaw,
> when told by doctors he would die
> if he refused meat.

Health is not an ingredient in the creation of paradise, but a benefit from it. It is humanity that is the blueprint for utopia. Without humanity, health is nothing but a sought-after fantasy that requires pursuing ever-increasing forms of violence (shark cartilage) in a vain attempt to overcome previous violence (surf and turf).

I've painted a pretty grim picture, perhaps, but all is not lost. Always remember the quintessential message of veganism (and even adopt it as your own): Treat all others as you would like all others to treat you. Upon doing so, look around; you may just find yourself in the paradise zone.

Hedonism and the Meaning of Life

Hedonism is a lifestyle of self-indulgence for one's own pleasure. On its face, it seems pretty good. But what if my pleasure is using your swimming pool ... or your wife ... or eating your dog (or your wife)? In the realm of hedonism, this is all perfectly acceptable and demonstrates that hedonism, paradoxically, cannot exist in paradise. While there is a basal appeal in the illusion of hedonism, it is simply a violent battlefield waiting to happen. Moreover, the more we indulge ourselves, the more unsatisfied we become.

You've probably heard the expression "It is better to give than to receive," and we've all experienced the profound joy in serving others. Giving provides a sense of fulfillment and meaning that is unattainable from getting. The greater the need we fill by giving, the greater the joy and sense of purpose derived. Try it for yourself and you will begin to see that service to others is the very meaning of life, and the more we help the most helpless, the greater our life.

Meat-eating society swallows the meaning of life three times a day, and then can't figure out why they can't find it.

The Enigma Explained

Most people love animals. Most people eat animals. Most people don't understand why our society is violent.

Talking Before Dinner, by Anthony R. Tag

"Pass the bread," Dad squirts
as beads of wine form on the clear plastic
table covering. The TV,
tired from Mom's dingy soap operas
and Dad's afternoon baseball snooze,
staggers through the news,
giving us only half the picture.
"That Jeffrey Dahmer is a monster," Mom chirps
as she pounds the bleeding steak on the counter.
"That man is disgusting," Dad burps.
"He deserves the electric chair."
Mom, shoving the bubbling crabs deep
into the boiling pot, closing the lid
on their clasping limbs, agrees.
"How can he watch people die, then eat them?"
"People like that have no respect for life," Dad answers.

Chapter 9

Humanity

"Non-violence leads to the highest ethics, which is the goal of all evolution. Until we stop harming all other living beings, we are still savages."   – Thomas Edison

Webster's *New World Dictionary* offers the following definition of the word "humanity": "The fact or quality of being humane; kindness, mercy, sympathy, etc." It is clear that turning a pig into a ham cannot come under the heading of humanity.

Practically every school in the country has courses in the humanities, and yet none of these have anything to do with humanity. It is sadly laughable. Humanities, as it is generally offered in most schools and universities, are courses in language and literature. For me, it is little wonder why our educated elite know literature extremely well but remain violent and inhumane. I can only hope that the following will one day become the essence of the curriculum in the humanities. Only when such a day arrives will society begin to understand and practice true humanity.

Animal Rights

"I am in favor of animal rights as well as human rights. That is the way of a whole human being."
                                                    – Abraham Lincoln

You may have seen those bumper stickers that bear slogans such as "Save the baby humans." This is a parody of slogans such as "Save the whales" and "Save the baby seals." Interestingly, it is a parody created by those who consider themselves to be "pro life," yet most pro-lifers eat meat. Putting that obvious hypocrisy aside for a moment, saving whales and baby seals is unnecessary. They don't need to be saved. They just need to be left alone, thank you very much. The bumper stickers imply we need to do something active, whereas we need to just leave them and their environment be.

Humanity is needed by all of us, for each of us, to benefit all of us. The term "animal rights" is highly misleading and is often propagated in a pejorative fashion. However, to fight for animal rights is based on a foundation of proper love and altruism. Whereas, for the most part, black people fight for black rights, women fight for women's rights, gays fight for gay rights, handicapped people fight for handicapped rights, and even adults who fight for the rights of abused children were often abused as children, nobody who fights for animal rights does so because they fear that they will be brought to slaughter. This fight is for justice, for love, for peace, for the Earth, and it is a fight based on altruism. It isn't even about rights at all; it is about curtailing cruelty and inhumanity and, in its place, building kindness, humanity and proper dominionship for all of God's creatures. Vegans may very well be the only completely altruistic people on the planet. Won't you join us?

> *"And there are the ideas of the future ... of freeing the slaves, of giving equality to women, [and] of ceasing to use flesh food."* — Leo Tolstoy

The term "animal rights" is misleading because it does nothing but ensure unending debate, just as we have done with all other civil rights: women's rights, black rights, gay rights, handicapped rights, children's rights, etc. It is not much more than another issue to throw onto the pile, which keeps society moving farther and farther away from truth (and, therefore, "rights" becomes a fallacious concept). However, animal rights and civil rights are (or should be) basic humanity; nothing more and nothing less. Nothing could be simpler or actualized more instantaneously.

Humanity is the recognition of the fact that all human-kind wants the very same thing, as does all animalkind. Proper love and humanity, animal rights, if you must, is the only foundation from which black rights, women's rights and any other civil rights can truly flourish. Rights and justice will never crystallize when selfishness is the motivation. When society aligns itself to these humanitarian principles, black rights and animal rights alike will be nonissues. The hypocrisy of the pyramid will be non-existent. Sovereignty of the individual will be honored above all else, and all creatures with a will to live will be respected and not denied their unalienable rights. Until such time as society embraces these principles, however, rights of any kind remain a vainly sought-after concept, and nothing more.

In the most simple yet most profound terms, animal rights is Humanities 101.

The Man Who Loves Animals

I know a man who says he loves animals. He really believes he does. Unfortunately, he is very much like millions of people around the world. I used to be a lot like him, too. I'll call this man Jonathan.

Jonathan loves dogs. They're wonderful to pet and play with, and he likes to keep them chained up outside for protection and security.

Jonathan loves deer. After all, they're beautiful creatures. So beautiful, in fact, that Jonathan has a nice big deer's head mounted on the wall in his living room.

Jonathan loves cows and pigs. He loves them so much he has given them new names: beef and pork.

Jonathan loves monkeys. Without them, upon whom would our scientists perform bizarre and cruel experiments?

Jonathan hasn't yet figured out how to love mice, so he buys mouse traps.

Jonathan sincerely believes he loves animals.

If animals could speak, which of them – the dog, the deer, the cow, the pig, the monkey, the mouse – would say they feel loved by Jonathan? With so much love like Jonathan's around, is it any wonder that the world is so brutal?

> *"I'm not a vegetarian because I love animals; I'm a vegetarian because I hate plants."* – A. Whitney Brown

Being humane, and loving animals (and people), means to care about what is good for them. It means to avoid exploiting them for one's own greed, gluttony, need for control over others and other wanton needs. It means to love them for who and what they are, not for what they can do for you. John F. Kennedy had a good premise, but even that was to serve his purposes. A minor variation on the same theme is called for: Ask not what God, His creatures and the world can do for you, ask what you can do for God, His creatures and the world. This is the basis of proper stewardship and dominionship over the planet.

Controlling Control

Where there is no humanity, love is likely to be dysfunctional. Jonathan's behavior shows love without humanity. In his case it is a love of having his way with animals. What Jonathan really loves is control. Would Jonathan love a dog he couldn't control? He'd probably just have it "put to sleep." The difference between loving behavior and the love of control is a key difference between humanity and brutality.

"A man who wants to control his animal passions easily does so if he controls his palate." –Mahatma Gandhi

Many people are devoid of humanity and express love dysfunctionally, just as Jonathan does. In the busy, dizzying modern world, children are more controlled than they are loved, so they learn that love means controlling others. Ergo, our love for others (people and animals) often manifests itself not unlike Jonathan's. Remember, dysfunctional love is replete with expectations *from* others. Humanity and proper love embraces the notion of service *to* others.

In an atmosphere of this control, proper love and humanity are largely absent. To make matters worse, when there is little or no love and humanity, children rebel and go out of control. Parents react by attempting not to love them, but to control them even more. We now have an inhumane world where most people have little or no self-control or individual sovereignty, but spend their lives attempting to control others. Children mimic what they see, and when you see an out-of-control child, you can bet the ranch there is an out-of-control adult nearby.

Self-control, or self-empowerment, if you prefer, is an extension of humanity and individual sovereignty. Learning self-control eliminates the need to control others. It comes from love of thyself, and you can only love others properly when you love yourself properly. And one who loves himself properly, one who is humane, cannot allow another to be killed, as much for his own comfort as for the comfort of the potential victim.

To offer love to another means being vulnerable, and that can seem scary, since being vulnerable can feel like giving up control. Cultivating vulnerability can seem like promoting weakness. On the contrary, it is the greatest strength of all. You reap what you sow.

Until people adhere to the principles of individual sovereignty, humanity remains, in the best of cases, abstract.

Give It To Me, Baby

Human beings have certain drives or innate desires that can guide us to a rewarding life, and they each may exist at different levels of consciousness. Food and sex are two that immediately come to mind. They are, to some degree, like emotions. They are tools that need to be used properly, but they can all be used improperly.

A less frequently discussed (and far less understood) drive is control. Just as we are all born with the drive to eat, we are all born with a drive to control; it's a necessary drive. Unfortunately, the vast majority of people – like Jonathan – never learn how to use this tool properly and, therefore, dysfunction is almost sure to follow. Like any drive, it will manifest itself one way or another, so we need to learn how to utilize it properly or trouble and dysfunction are the result.

Used properly, the control drive manifests as self-control. We must learn how to control our thoughts and actions or we become dysfunctional and spend our lives attempting to control others. With a lack of self-control, you will have a world of control-hungry regimes, man over man, man over animal, the strong over the weak.

"Be gentle to all and stern with yourself"
                                        –Saint Teresa of Avila

Self Control: A Test

Sit down in a nice quiet room, get comfortable and close your eyes. For two minutes try to think about absolutely nothing. See if you can remain alert while keeping your mind completely still.

Difficult, isn't it? If you've tried the test, you now realize just how little self-control you really have. If you controlled your legs as well as you control your mind, you probably wouldn't be able to get out of bed.

Pursue methods of gaining self-control, such as Stepping Back or meditation, as this is the key to attaining and maintaining paradise. It's one thing to control your actions and become vegan because you read a book that seemed to make sense. But what happens when another book comes out with a persuasive argument to the contrary? Self-control of the mind will enable you to reach truths on your own, without the need for this or any other book.

Gain self-control and you will have man over himself, entirely over himself and over only himself. You will have individual sovereignty and no need for regimes, parliaments or Congress. The need for control of others becomes nonexistent because the tool is being used properly. In an environment of self-control, we will each be our own masters to pursue life, liberty and happiness and let all others do the same. In other words ... vegan.

The Value Of Life

Meat eaters who have never even considered life beyond their own indoctrination think vegans are so silly to equate the life of a human with the life of a chicken or a cow or a mouse or a monkey. People who eat animals think that a chicken is "worth" about one dollar per pound.

Firstly, life is part of nature; money isn't. This, in itself, could be the basis of a book – or three. Secondly, the concept that a chicken's life has a monetary value is not unlike the concept of slavery, in which you could buy a black man for money. It's not even that far from Nazi Germany killing Jews because in the Nazis' minds Jews actually had a negative worth. It cost money to get rid of these people. It is clear that anyone who kills a human being or owns another human being sullies himself. People who put a monetary value on life, any life, also sully themselves.

Animal eaters look at life through very tainted eyes. To them, a chicken's life is worth one dollar per pound and, therefore, they see vegans as bringing down the value of human life to this level. But the reality is something *very* different. To apply a cash value to any life diminishes the real, inherent value of all life to the level of money. Money is inherently valueless. Conversely, to uphold the actual, inherent value of any life (far beyond that of money) uplifts all life to a level far greater than our society now places even on human life. Wisdom, born out of truth and enhanced by instinct, tells us in no uncertain terms that the life of all creatures is every bit as important and "valuable" to them as our life is to us. This is humanity.

The animal eater sees a human life as being worth more than the life of a chicken – a relative worth. Therefore, part of the problem is the desire for money and control (one and the same), and part of the problem is the belief in the pyramidal scheme of superiority over others. The animal eater not only sees the life of an animal as worth less than the life of a man, but sees the life of Tom Smith as worth less than the life of Tom Cruise. If you don't believe me, who do you think would get a kidney transplant first? To an animal-eating society, which is a society that lives according to the philosophy of the pyramids, all life has a value relative only to the one under it, thereby denigrating all life.

Conversely, however, a vegan lifestyle upholds the sanctity of all life truly equally, thereby elevating the value of life to a plateau light years above anything to do with money.

Don't be confused by control-hungry flesh eaters who assign a price for flesh and then cite monetary values as a basis that humans are "worth more than animals." They use the fallacious post hoc ergo propter hoc as fact. Monetary value of any life is complete, absolute and categorical nonsense. One being worth more than another is a dangerous absurdity that lives in the darkness of The Big Lie. To an animal eater, all life is sullied. To a vegan, all life is sacred. If any man, woman or child wants to live in a world where life is truly respected and sacred, then he or she must be vegan. All life is sacred in paradise.

"Life is sacred, that is to say, it is the supreme value, to which all other values are subordinate."
–Albert Einstein

Quit Talking Nonsense

When some men get together they may talk about how much smarter they are than women. What is really going on here is a lack of understanding between groups. In reality, are women less smart than men, or is it that men aren't smart enough to understand women? People often justify their cruel ways bestowed upon animals in the same way.

Every day I hear people say things like, "Animals aren't smart enough to communicate," or, "It's okay to eat animals because they don't feel it." Animals are sentient creatures with a will to live, advanced communication abilities and an observable intellect. Whales, for example, have a vocabulary at least as complex as man's. Dolphins are now used regularly to help in the treatment of disabled people, as they can sense what is going on in our bodies. Dogs are being used to sniff out cancer in humans. Gorillas have actually learned sign language, which means they must be smarter than us in some ways, as we have been unable to learn their language. It's not that animals aren't smart enough or sentient enough, but actually that we are not yet smart enough to understand them and to simply appreciate and embrace our differences. It is our dulled perceptions that don't comprehend their methods of communication or feeling. Unfortunately, once people develop a taste for meat, they don't really want to "un-dull" themselves and tune in. All of this aside, even if they are less smart, so what? If my IQ is higher than yours, does that give me license to be inhumane to you?

Slowly, however, even meat eaters are learning the wonder of nonhuman animals, and in recent years products such as dolphin-safe tuna have become more popular. As well-meaning as this is, it's a lot like attempting to get somewhere and each time always traveling half the distance – you'll never get there. Even though dolphin-safe tuna is a step in the right direction, many dolphins and other sea creatures are still killed in the nets. And besides all that, what about the tuna?

Cutting Through The Smoke

A smoke screen is something said or done to conceal or mislead. A few years ago, Disney released the live action version of _101 Dalmatians_. This is the story of a villainous woman named Cruella De Vil who is in pursuit of the spotted canines so she can make a coat from their coats. This is the essence of what makes her evil. Kids, being very connected to their innate humanity and instinct, love animals. Someone who is looking to harm animals easily becomes an antagonist, and you could hear children booing Cruella in theaters all over the world. McDonald's was a huge participant in the promotion of the Disney movie and offered _101 Dalmatians_ toys and merchandising through their restaurants. The fictional Cruella, who was looking to kill a few dogs, is small-time compared to McDonald's, which is actually responsible for brutalizing and murdering millions upon millions upon millions of fish, chickens and cows (and people, from heart disease, cancer, etc.). Kids were able to go into a McDonald's restaurant and order a Happy Meal complete with a _101 Dalmatians_ toy. After swallowing the flesh of a violently murdered animal, they'd go home with their toy, all the while believing they were the animal world's best friends.

Smoke Screen #1,073,452

During the end credits of movies such as *101 Dalmatians*, the producers feel compelled to add a disclaimer that reads: "No animals were harmed during the making of this movie." This reassures viewers who may be sensitive about animal welfare that the movie was only make-believe. That's great except for just one small thing. What about the countless animals that were killed to feed the cast and crew?

Humanity must not be make-believe, unless we want paradise to be make-believe.

It's Raining Cats And Dogs

Instinctively and innately we are a world of animal lovers. In the United States alone, there are well over one hundred million dogs and cats. It is difficult to come to the realization that owning "pets" out of a love of animals is backwards logic. A good example of backwards logic is banging your head against a wall because it feels good when you stop.

People point to their dog or cat as a token of their loving spirit toward animals, then they go to the refrigerator and pull out some variety of animal flesh to prepare the evening meal. On the road to paradise, this is road block # 2,000,000.

Additionally, we murder millions of other animals to feed our dogs and cats. Why are chickens, pigs and cows less worthy of love than dogs and cats? Love of animals, you say? Road block # 2,000,001, I say.

Some of the worst perpetrators of animal brutality are actually dog and cat breeders. They love to talk about how much they love animals; that's why they're breeders. Does the breeder's love extend to any of the millions of homeless animals (since there are already too many dogs and cats) that wander the streets until they're caught and euthanized in animal shelters? At any given moment there are hundreds of thousands of homeless dogs and cats locked up in tiny steel cages awaiting execution. These are our "best friends." What do we do? Breed more. Roadblock # 2,000,002.

Why do we feel we need to "own" an animal to show the world (and ourselves) that we are animal lovers? All animals are, or should be, entitled to love and to individual sovereignty. Murdering millions upon millions of cows and pigs, etc., to feed dogs and cats is not love of animals of any meaningful kind. This is more backwards logic. We first breed them to satisfy our own selfish whims and then insist it is natural that these artificially created "pets" eat other animals.

When we stop eating animals we develop a very special kinship with all living creatures and may not have the need to have a pet to express or experience our love. Love will be omnipresent. Love exists and will be apparent every and any time we are in the presence of another. One species' fear of another will be replaced by respect, appreciation and kinship. Breeding animals to create tokens of "love of animals" will be rightly seen as brutal, selfish folly.

I'm not in any way suggesting you give up the animals you live with now. They are certainly entitled to life and love. However, if we are motivated out of love, we must curtail the breeding and owning of animals, especially carnivorous animals. We will all be better for it.

Fortunately, dogs are actually omnivores and will eat nearly anything given to them. In fact, a vegan diet is completely healthy for them. Cats, on the other hand, are mostly carnivorous and seem to have a nutritional requirement for taurine that a vegan diet may not supply. However, there are vegan cat foods on the market that are supplemented with synthetic taurine, which, ironically, is the same synthetic taurine that is added to meat-based cat foods, as even these do not provide this essential amino acid. If you have a dog and you love animals you should immediately begin feeding it a vegan diet (slowly transitioning over the course of a week or two). If you have cats and you love animals, you should immediately mix their regular food half and half with a quality vegan cat food. Then you should read the book *Obligate Carnivore*, by Jed Gillen, or *Vegetarian Cats & Dogs*, by James A. Peden, after which you will be enlightened enough to further curtail, and eventually eliminate, meat for all your cats and dogs; for their good, your good and for love of all humanity.

Breeders are responsible for enormous amounts of animal suffering. Do not buy animals from breeders or retail pet stores, which get their animals from breeders. This is not love, but the outright destruction of love. Rather, go to an animal shelter and give a home to an animal that doesn't have one. Take it in to your home, make it permanent, treat it like you would like to be treated, and feed it a humane, vegan food. This is love.

Some people ask what we should do with all the cows in the world if we and our companion animals stopped eating them. The answer is, we should stop breeding them too (and yes, care for the ones that are already here).

Unconventional Humanity

True humanity cannot be thought of or referred to in conventional terms, because there is no real humanity in conventional terms. True humanity is a behavior of love, respect and compassion for all who reside on our planet, with complete and categorical disregard for any of the conventional paradigms (finances, sexism, racism, speciesism). It is only upon this foundation that a decent, humanitarian society can be properly built. Meatism is violence whereas veganism is humanity, and the very nature of paradise mandates that we be vegan.

Chapter 10

Peace, Freedom...
& UFOs?

Freedom should not be viewed as a political right granted by governments, rather, freedom should be inextricably woven into the basic doctrine of all humanity for all humanity. The most wonderful aspect of the United States, for example, is its alignment with this philosophy, as enshrined in the Constitution, and it is this alignment that makes this country such a powerful force. However, this power is not generated by the government but by the people, people who hold freedom to be one of the highest principles of humanity. Unfortunately, as much as we believe in freedom, society will never know its true power until freedom is practiced as a behavior and not denied to any of the Earth's inhabitants.

To have true freedom we must not deny true freedom to any living creature, and for one to practice freedom in the truest sense of the word, one must be vegan. To create even some semblance of paradise, a world in which there is harmony, peace and freedom must be an integral part of the lives of all sentient creatures. We cannot properly claim we are in favor of freedom while we take away the freedom of those weaker than ourselves. We cannot kill, eat or experiment on animals and know true freedom ourselves. It is not possible.

"This is a world of compensation; and he who would be no slave must consent to have no slave. Those who deny freedom to others deserve it not for themselves, and, under a just God, cannot long retain it."

– Abraham Lincoln

Close Encounter Of The Fourth Kind

Let's say that one day a UFO finally did the logical thing – it landed in New York City for everyone to see instead of in the middle of Wyoming. Now, let's say these extraterrestrial creatures despaceship (that's alien for deplane) and our top government officials are there to greet them. If these aliens were capable of immediately vaporizing our planet, the government, seeking to get on their good side, would offer to have them over to the White House for an incredible intergalactic party.

But let's consider another scenario. What would happen if these alien creatures couldn't vaporize the planet and, moreover, were not even strong enough to defend themselves? We all assume they would be quite strong since they are capable of space travel, but let's say for whatever reason they are not. Let's also say that we were not able to establish any type of understandable communication with them. In this case, would our government officials offer to have them over to the White House for that dinner party? Of course not. Those types of parties are reserved for those with the potential to be formidable opponents – the super-rich, the powerful, heads of state, etc. Our peace-loving aliens would be taken to a laboratory somewhere to be experimented upon. Since they can't speak out or defend themselves, the scientists could and would do just about anything to them. Then, at the end of each day, when the scientists are getting ready to go home, they would put these meek creatures (those still alive after the day's experiments) in locked cages so they couldn't roam off and "hurt themselves."

Is it any wonder the aliens are so elusive and only go to Wyoming at three o'clock in the morning?

If they can beat us up, we wine and dine them. If we can beat them up, we do. This might-over-right philosophy isn't just the practice of uneducated street punks, this is the societal elite.

> *"There is something so very dreadful, so satanic in tormenting those who have never harmed us, and who cannot defend themselves, who are utterly in our power, who have weapons neither of offense or defense, that none but the very hardened persons can endure the thought of it."* — Cardinal Newman

Let Freedom Ring

If we believe in freedom, we must be willing to come to its defense. Further, we may even need to fight for it, for ourselves and, equally, for the freedom of others. If we don't, there may be nobody left to fight for us when our time comes. And besides all of this, upholding freedom is a basic responsibility of each and every member of the human race.

As members of the human race who embrace truth, justice, life and liberty, we must take a look at the freedom and liberty being denied to any and all of the Earth's inhabitants, and we must be careful to guard against any complicity where these vital elements to humanity are denied. We must be vegan.

> *I am the voice of the voiceless;*
> *through me the dumb shall speak.*
> *Till the deaf world's ear be made to hear*
> *the cry of the wordless weak.*

And I am my brother's keeper,
and I will fight his fight;
and speak the word for beast and bird
till the world shall set things right.
　　　　　　　　– Excerpted from *Voice of the Voiceless,*
　　　　　　　　　　　by Ella Wheeler Wilcox

If we want peace, if we believe in freedom, if we believe in humanity, and if we are humane beings, we must recognize that might over right has no place in our world or in our lives. We must embrace freedom and humanity for all the Earth's inhabitants, and do so notwithstanding the old habits of The Big Lie, the thirst for blood and sociopathic denial. Choosing to embrace freedom and humanity means meat must be abolished from our lives. We will then, and only then, witness humanity and freedom flourish upon the Earth. Then, and only then, will we *all* live free with absolute right to life, liberty and the pursuit of happiness, as originally intended by our Creator.

Freedom Director

There should be a person or persons (call it a government if you must, though it is quite the opposite) whose sole job it would be to sustain and protect all freedom. In any cases where freedom is being denied they would develop and implement strategies to correct it forthwith. This job would not have any other functions or abilities, nor would it give a select few authority over others. Its sole function would be to ensure authority over none. This job should not and must not be political unless we want freedom to be political.

Every inhabitant of the planet must be allowed to pursue the life given to them. This is the only way to move forward on the road to paradise.

"In all the round world of utopia there is no meat."
— H.G. Wells

Factory Farms

Grazing land is becoming scarce on our planet, largely due to the meat industry, so enter factory farms. This high-tech approach to supplying animal products to millions of people are enclosed warehouse-type buildings that are run truly like factories, and they take the denial of freedom to new lows. They are a marvel of technology — and brutality. In fact, putting the animals forced to live in those appalling conditions out of their daily misery by murdering them can almost seem humane.

> *"Modern cowboys no longer run five hundred head on ten thousand acres of prairie. Today, they are more likely to run ten thousand head on five acres of concrete."*   — *May All Be Fed*, by John Robbins

Without any compassion or decency whatsoever (since these animals are now nothing more than products), many animals spend their entire lives in these factory farms. Cows, pigs, chickens and others who were meant to live free — free to roam, free to socialize and play — are now raised in cages so small they can't even turn around. In the name of profits, the conditions under which these animals are forced to live are horrific beyond comprehension.

Some time ago a radio station made an offer of several thousand dollars to anyone who could live under similar conditions to that of an animal in a factory farm. No one was able to claim the money, even though it was only for forty-eight hours. Just imagine having an itch and not being able to scratch it (try it sometime), not being able to sit or lie down comfortably, not being able to move. Imagine no natural light and no natural order of day and night, only timed intervals of light for feeding purposes. Imagine not being able to get into a natural position for eating. The food is just placed under your nose because you can't reach it any other way. Imagine not being able to groom yourself or socialize (although you would be so miserable that you probably wouldn't want to socialize). Imagine the horrible smells and sounds of all the others forced to live the same excruciating way. Imagine being forced to urinate and defecate where you lie, onto a grated steel floor so your waste can fall below onto a fellow sufferer, just as the droppings of another sufferer above fall onto you. This is your life, forever, or at least until they decide to slaughter you. This is part of a society that believes in freedom?

Anybody who eats meat and animal products is directly participating in the cruelty, brutality and torture of animals that have no freedom – none. Take a moment right now to really imagine being born into immediate and permanent suffering.

The best day for these animals is the day after they die, because they are no longer suffering. Eating and using animal products is taking away freedom, creating enormous suffering, destroying the planet, and violating everything good, just and decent. This is the belief in freedom devoid of the behavior of freedom. Without customers for their products, the factory farms would cease to exist. Your call.

Free Range Ideas

Some people attempt to incorporate their old meat-eating habits with a New Age concept of "free range" meat (or eggs or milk). Free range products come from animals that were allowed to, as the name implies, roam free instead of being locked up in cages. Free range products attempt to curtail animal suffering while still exploiting and murdering them.

And while the concept of free range implies we can have our eggs and eat them too, that concept is a myth.

When billions of people crave these products there is, in reality, no way to adequately supply them by allowing animals to have their natural freedom. (This should be telling us something.) Nonetheless, a few sensitive meat eaters attempt to meld two mutually exclusive ideas – freedom and exploitation. Then, the sheer volume of demand forces that there be no freedom.

Oftentimes, people become vegetarian believing that the production of milk and eggs isn't harming animals. In my personal process of becoming vegan I, too, was first a vegetarian. I would say to myself that if I kept chickens in my backyard and took very good care of them and they laid eggs, then it would, therefore, be a symbiotic, or mutually supporting, relationship; and it would be perfectly okay to eat their eggs. And while this may seem true at a shallow level, there is a deeper truth.

Firstly, if I continue to eat eggs with this philosophy in mind and then I go out of town and stay in a hotel, I would probably order eggs for breakfast. After all, I am an egg eater. The eggs at the hotel, however, are not coming from a symbiotic relationship. So I'll overlook this "one time."

Secondly, there is no true way for the chickens of the planet to humanely and symbiotically supply breakfast to billions of hungry people. Developing a taste for eggs will cause demand to rise. When demand exceeds supply, something must be done to increase that supply. And there, my friends, goes any real concept of humane treatment of chickens. Planet Earth simply cannot support enough free range chickens to supply billions of hungry people, hence factory farms. By you eating free range, somebody else can't, and, therefore, there is a chicken (many, actually) somewhere that *must* be kept in a tiny cage because *you* chose to eat an egg.

Thirdly, what do we do with all the male chickens who take up room and eat but obviously don't lay eggs? The reality is they are systematically killed – usually suffocated in plastic bags.

Fourthly, while the concept of chickens happily roaming around my backyard is pleasing, the reality is I have never had even one chicken in my backyard. The concept of free range is simply the justification process of a mind that strives for humanity with a habit that couldn't care less. Free range beef, free range chicken, free range eggs, free range milk are mythical and, at best, a slippery slope from freedom to torture. True freedom requires veganism.

Make Love Not War

Perhaps even General George S. Patton might agree that antiwar activists have an innocent charm to them. Well, maybe not Patton. But the "innocence" of these people is also naïve, as they are equally responsible for war. They will lie down in the street chanting, "No more innocent bloodshed," then strategize their next protest over a chicken sandwich or hamburger lunch. If we trace war and violence all the way back to their origins, we will see that the first act of violence was killing animals. Even today, violent adults were often abused as children, and as abused children they turned around and began the cycle all over again by abusing animals, and then, over time, people.

If you really want to be pro peace, job number one is to stop the bloodshed, the blood which *you* spill. You must be vegan before you can work for no more wars. There are absolutely no politicians, even those who are purportedly pro peace, who can ever accomplish peace while they participate in the bloodshed of others.

We can look back thousands of years to accurately see that there have always been those who destroy peace by attempting to take freedom away from others. Ironically, therefore, wars for freedom (and peace) may sometimes be necessary.

To behave in accordance with the principles of freedom, one must be vegan. To be an animal lover, one must be vegan. To be good, just and decent, one must be vegan. To be an environmentalist, one must be vegan. To be truthful, loving and healthy, one must be vegan. To understand the meaning of life, one must be vegan.

To walk the road to paradise, to walk in the path of God, one *must* be vegan.

Chapter 11

Religion

In my personal and lengthy journey of stepping back in my quest for truth I came to a very hard question that I struggled with for a long time. Though each and every part of my journey had merit, no single answer bound it all together; until that one day when I opened, or rather reopened, the Bible.

The question: If there is a God, if God is about love, if love is about veganism, and if God wants mankind to be vegan, why hasn't he expressly and in absolutely, positively no uncertain terms told us so? I struggled with that question for longer than I care to remember.

I wondered about man's evil nature. I truly felt that man isn't so much evil by intention, but rather by misinformation and misguidance. So, then, why wouldn't God simply tell us to be vegan, since surely all good and decent men would follow His word? I must confess that I even wondered why God wouldn't simply appear at the Super Bowl halftime show and tell the millions of viewers to be vegan.

The Holy Bible was written in three languages and then, over time, translated into over two thousand more. The Bible is the best-selling book in the world, with roughly 6.5 billion copies printed through the ages. In the Western World we are almost always within a few feet of one. The

Bible is even more accessible than the Super Bowl halftime show, and there is not a man, woman or child on Planet Earth who cannot lay their hands and set their eyes upon it.

One serendipitous day, I (re)opened the Bible and there, on **PAGE ONE**, was the answer. It was legible, it was clear, it was in black and white, and in no uncertain terms it was the basis for human behavior as set forth by our Creator:

> *"And God said: 'Let the Earth put forth grass, herb yielding seed, and fruit-tree bearing fruit after its kind, wherein is the seed thereof, upon the Earth.' And it was so. And the Earth brought forth grass, herb yielding seed after its kind, and tree bearing fruit, wherein is the seed thereof, after its kind; and God saw that it was good."*
> (Genesis 1:11-12)

This passage comes immediately after God created the world. Then, immediately after God created man, comes the following:

> *"And God said: 'Behold, I have given you every herb yielding seed, which is upon the face of all the Earth, and every tree, in which is the fruit of a tree yielding seed – to you it shall be for food ..."*   (Genesis 1:29)

Page one of the Bible has been printed *6.5 billion times*. It was crystal clear. God did give us the answer. Then I thought maybe He should just say it one more time, and then I laughed. How many times must it be said? Is 6.5 billion times not enough? You just need to open your eyes and wipe the blood away to see it. Any more questions?

Blind? Or Unwilling to See?

It is astounding that religious people can read that passage from the Bible, go to church or temple once or twice a week, and then go home, eat a hot dog and say they believe in God.

Then, if asked about this passage, they'll say something like, "Well, it doesn't say we can't eat animals." Folks, the Bible doesn't say, "Thou shalt not fly airplanes into buildings," either. It was just simply that God hadn't foreseen man's astoundingly vile abilities. It is much like a parent giving a car to his sixteen-year-old-child. Must the parent tell the child specifically everything that the child must not do with the car? You must not use the car to rob banks. You must not use the car to run people over, etc. Such a premise is an absurdity. You create a child, raise the child and hope that the child has developed a level of responsibility so that such absurd instructions need not be given, since it would be impossible to cover every misuse.

How can religion routinely and summarily skip right over God's earliest directive? In no uncertain terms, this directive tells us what He has given us to eat in His "good" world. If any man or woman on the planet chooses to deny this first truth of our existence and then puts into place a lifestyle contrary to this truth and justifies it through their entire lives, they don't change this truth, because truth remains truth.

The literal truth is, according to the Bible, God didn't say don't eat pigs – green pigs, white pigs, dancing pigs, short pigs. Nor did he say don't eat fish – big fish, little fish, singing fish, polka-dotted fish. A more important, literal truth is, God *did* say, "Thou shalt not kill."

Any more questions?

Closing In On The Source

Of course, in later passages the Bible refers to eating meat. But if all the Bible is the word of God, how can it contain such a stark contradiction? Is God a hypocrite? Page one of the Bible shows people how to behave in accordance with paradise. The other couple of thousand pages show us the nefarious confusion and hypocrisy once meat enters the equation. Stepping back all the way to the beginning of existence, to Creation, if you like, makes clear the need for veganism in a paradise.

The Bible is largely a tool of religion and before an enlightened discussion about God can take place, we must first discuss religion and understand that there is a difference between the two. Earlier, we discussed the important difference between patriotism and freedom. Patriotism can be a dangerous facade, whereas freedom is what actually matters. Religion is a lot like patriotism, and, in fact, more people embrace religion than they do God. This presents several problems. We are a world so focused on the dogma, customs and traditions of our individual religions, and, therefore, so enamored by religion itself, that we are willing to blindly follow it. All the while, we haven't stopped to consider the meaningful substance behind it all and whether religion is really the best vehicle to our desired destination. God and religion are not the same.

As with patriotism, religion facilitates self-serving wars of every kind and magnitude, which accomplishes nothing but more war. Islamic extremists call the perpetrators of 9/11 martyrs because they believed that by killing as many "infidels" as possible while killing themselves, they would go to paradise. We know this is absurd and has nothing to do with God, because we know that God is love, and blowing up people is not love. This is religion.

Christianity, Judaism and Islam, for example, tell us that it is okay to kill others and eat their dead bodies. It should be equally clear that this is not love either. Violating someone's individual sovereignty, killing them, is not love. Killing animals is not proper love and cannot have anything to do with God. This, again, is religion. Religion and God are not the same. In fact, in many ways they are mutually exclusive. We must unlearn what religions have corrupted us with for eons, that religion and God are the same. They are not.

"A missionary was walking in Africa when he heard the ominous padding of a lion behind him.

'Oh, Lord,' prayed the missionary, 'grant in thy goodness that the lion walking behind me is a good, Christian lion.'

And then, in the silence that followed, the missionary heard the lion praying too: 'Oh, Lord,' he prayed, 'we thank thee for the food which we are about to receive.'"
– Cleveland Amory

Who Are the Wild Animals?

In the earliest parts of the Bible, when the Earth was a paradise (Eden), there was God, man and animals. We were given dominion over the animals and, therefore, it was our job to be their caretaker. Instead, we began eating them, dividing us from each other, from them and from God, and setting into motion an altered reality from what was originally intended.

Since most of us have experience interacting with dogs and cats, consider this example. Dogs and cats that are raised with love and kindness are usually kind and loving. Dogs and cats that are mistreated are usually quite nasty and unhappy. Further, dogs and cats that aren't loved or socialized at all become virtually "wild animals." Feral cats and dogs (and even feral children) are every bit as wild as lions, tigers and bears. Oh, my.

However, most of us still pretend that lions, tigers and bears are naturally wild animals. Then, the humans who choose to eat meat often point to the wild animals that do the same thing "naturally" as justification for doing so. Isn't it just possible – even probable – that *we* have created these wild animals? Our lack of love, truth and service to others has created chasms (seemingly natural, yet actually man-made) between *all* who would otherwise reside together in paradise. We readily acknowledge that dogs and cats to which we are neglectful to one degree or another become wild animals. Conversely, those to whom we are kind and loving are our companions. Mankind, meat-eating mankind that is, refuses to acknowledge the truth that all animals are capable of love, kindness, kinship and companionship, and that it is our neglect and mismanagement of our dominion-ship that is facilitating this misplaced belief in the first place. Yet, how grand (almost incomprehensible) it would be to be kin with all existence.

We must start closing the gaps. The first step is to become vegan. You can then say to all existence, " You need not fear me. I am your friend." Then, as we progress, we must do what true friends do – care for each other. If we all do this, the history books will show it wasn't the lions, tigers and bears that were the wild animals. As we build bridges back to those *we've* abandoned, we may very well find all bridges become viable once again.

Even if all the Bible is an entire fabrication, and God is as real as Bugs Bunny, then being vegan is still curative. Being vegan replaces viciousness with humanity. Veganism makes the world a kinder and more loving place. This is truth. (With or without the Bible, with or without religion, even with or without God.)

Do I Dare Talk About <u>Him</u>?

Most people in the world believe in some form of God. The Jews have theirs, the Christians have theirs, the Buddhists, Hindus and Muslims have theirs. People of certain Eastern religions try to reach God through the self, while others in the West look externally. In each case, the personification of the concept varies, but the essence is utterly similar. That essence is love.

All sentient creatures have the emotion of love, call it a soul if you like, and that is, or should be, the direct connection to God. However, if you don't utilize proper love, you place a roadblock, or veil, between you and God, no matter how much religion you may have.

So let's consider for a moment the idea taught and condoned by religions that animals were put here by a loving God for us to kill and eat. God is a good, just, enlightened and loving power who creates animals with the same fight or flight hormones as us and senses including, but not limited to, pain, fear and survival instincts. Creating an animal for the very purpose of exploiting these senses by killing and eating them is downright sadistic, diametrically opposed to our notion of God. Religion's tenets and God's tenets are mutually exclusive.

> *"There may be some foolish people in the future who will say that I permitted meat-eating and that I partook of meat myself, but meat-eating I have not permitted to anyone, I do not permit, I will not permit meat-eating in any form in future, in any manner and in any place. It is unconditionally prohibited for all."* – The Buddha

If God is sadistic, perhaps people ought to reconsider who they worship, since worshiping a sadistic God can only help to create a sadistic society. I am certainly not implying that I think God is sadistic; quite the contrary. I believe that no matter what form this power takes, it is a good, just, enlightened and loving force. But a good, just, enlightened and loving force cannot create fear and pain for the purpose of exploiting it, as this is the epitome of sadism and evil. Inflicting pain on others is how meat eaters live their lives, then they project this nonsense onto God as one of His attributes in an attempt to justify their own behavior. It is this irreconcilable dichotomy that holds the beginnings of all hypocrisy.

> *"I tremble for my species, when I reflect that God is just."*
>   – Thomas Jefferson

Therefore, if God is, as we believe, good, just, enlightened and loving, He, in no way, shape or form could have possibly created sentient creatures for the end purpose of feeling pain, isolation, terror, etc.; in other words, for being killed and eaten. These faculties are part of sentient life so that one can protect oneself from hazards to life, not just so one can feel terror and pain as the end result. That's why humans feel pain and that's why nonhuman animals feel pain. Pain is a defense mechanism to avoid further pain and danger. It is one of the simplest truths to recognize if the subject matter is approached truthfully and objectively. Yet this is not how most religions approach the subject of God, or eating meat.

One of the most troubling concepts to grasp in stepping back to find the real solutions to it all is that religions may actually play a key role in keeping us from our God. It is wildly fascinating that many religions teach that Satan (evil personified) tries to work evil ways at times by appearing as an angel. If such a force exists, how devilishly brilliant of it to create religion and then use it to instill the belief that this is the "good" path for man to follow. Yet, in actuality, this path, created by evil, takes us farther and farther away from compassion, enlightenment and love – and God. This religion, Satan's angel, is the antithesis of God.

> *"Hide in plain sight."*
>   – Unknown

It's Halftime – Religion 21, God 3

Theology, the study of God, holds veganism as an ideal. This is not surprising, since God created man to be vegan. But theology is usually overseen by meat-eating religion, and the business entities known as "religions" have little to do with God (other than claiming a connection). Religion is about religion, an entity unto itself for its own purposes. As always, a lot of it has to do with money, and money has its roots in meat and in creating ownership of others. This is the antithesis of all that God represents – truth, love, individual sovereignty, etc. God has nothing whatsoever to do with money. God is about truth and love. Truth and love are about a vegan way of living.

In paradise, the environment of love, we *all* have paradise – and love. Christianity encourages the eating of fish on Fridays and Islam tells its adherents that paradise can exist for one at another's expense, with both meat and slaves available in the next world. So paradise for whom, exactly? The very basis of paradise within the context of this philosophy is an impossibility, and can aptly serve as a case study in how *not* to create a paradise. This philosophy does not encompass proper love and is, therefore, a dysfunctional and self-sabotaging process of pursuing paradise, which only serves to create the very violence that prevents the actualization of paradise.

How can any religion that is supposedly about spreading love not denounce the killing of *any* of God's creatures?

> "Re-examine all you have been told, dismiss what insults your soul."   – Walt Whitman

You Shall Have No Other Gods Before Me

Man's pyramidal philosophies create many intermediaries, such as governments, churches and even other people.

Individual sovereignty, on the other hand, allows mankind the direct connection to God, devoid of the intermediaries God has prohibited. Sovereignty of nations and churches makes nearly impossible that direct connection we are supposed to have. Religion is like a real estate agent, in that a real estate agent needs the buyer and seller to *not* know each other in order to make his commission. If you wanted to buy your best friend's house, and your best friend wanted to sell you his house, would you call a real estate agent?

Because God is absent in the presence of things ungodly, such as eating meat, religion can flourish. God cannot actively participate in a world that eats meat, as this is ungodly. God clearly intended for mankind to be vegan. If mankind were vegan, we would know God directly and, thus, have no real use for religion. With this real and direct connection to God, what would be the point of religion? Isn't it necessary, then, that religion, in order to continue, needs people to continue eating meat?

To put it another way, if you eat meat, you lose your connection to God, then religion steps in and tells you their version of an abstract paradise, and that your ticket there is to follow their rules, which they say are God's rules. If you don't follow these rules, the God of love will punish you. Are you dizzy yet?

Pursue truth.

Mankind having an actual relationship with God would render religion defunct. The way for you to develop a direct relationship with God is to first be vegan. It is also the way to allow others to do the same. It is only in this loving, vegan era that God can logically and naturally become manifest. In actuality, religions should be delighted about this prospect. However, they only came about once God removed himself from meat-eating man, and it was (and is) very easy for religions to step in and make you believe that they represent God, since God is no longer around or directly involved to dispute this. Besides, God is not a debater. God is God. Religions need you to eat God's animals, an evil practice, because in doing so, they can stay in existence. Are these religions truly about connecting you to God? Hardly. Religions are a monumental fortress lying squarely across the road to paradise.

There are even religions that have convoluted dietary rules that govern how to kill and eat animals. Some say the kosher dietary laws are God's laws for murdering animals. As if this wasn't absurd enough, these laws are some of the most heinous – the animals must be fully conscious while having their throats cut.

> *"If animals believe in God, then the devil would look like a human being."*   – Isaac Bashevis Singer

Any religion that sets forth a belief that God has issued procedures on how to murder His sentient animals is nothing more than a primrose path to hell. The Koran states that God (Allah) is "most merciful." Most merciful for whom, exactly? What constitutes a paradise for Muslims is a hell for animals. Christianity wants its adherents to believe that Jesus Christ, an all-loving God, murdered fish, his own sentient creatures, and fed them to people who were needy. Did the fish not need their lives? Do *you* really want to perpetuate this absurdity, this dysfunction, this hell on Earth? An all-loving, merciful God who ordains the perpetual suffering of others is neither loving nor merciful. This is not God at all. This is religion.

Fortunately, we can very easily know God if mankind lives up to its potential and responsibility, and behaves as though it were God, since we are created in His image. However, that doesn't mean having your way with people (and animals). God does not force his way upon people, as that is ungodly. God is pure and proper love. Give and receive it and you can begin to know God. In fact, love is what connects all who reside on this planet, as does the suffering brought about by the lack of it. It is impossible to give and receive proper love while eating God's creatures.

God has given you the gift of choice. You can choose any path you like. No one should take that choice away from you. But choice is a responsibility. Making the *right* choice is an even bigger responsibility. We are all in your hands, and vice versa. Do you want your hands eaten?

The Lord Works In Mysterious Ways ... Not!

Being a product of God and, therefore, having a soul, people are innately spiritual. However, there is a very good reason why there is so much discontentment with religions. Many religions seem to enjoy interpreting God's supposed word. Yet, because many times they aren't really offering the true word of God, and therefore can't find an answer that rings true, they will resort to the all-too-familiar cop-out of, "Well, the Lord works in mysterious ways." While religions may, in fact, work in very mysterious ways, God absolutely does not. God does not work through riddles, puzzles or cryptograms. When a religious leader makes statements that we instinctively know are not true (even if intellectually we don't know the correct answer), we are bound to feel uneasiness and discontentment. The Big Lie can conceal the truth but it cannot change the truth, and, therefore, one's instincts are one's own best defense. Be careful of anyone or anything that tells you the Lord works in mysterious ways.

A) God is good, just, enlightened and loving.

B) Killing is the antithesis of goodness, justice, enlightenment and love.

C) Therefore ... well, if you like puzzles, then you complete the syllogism.

"Every green herb for food" means every green herb for food, and "Thou shalt not kill" means thou shalt not kill. What part of this do meat-eating religions not understand?

For those who want to see the truth, it is very clear. Any religion that doesn't truly follow the word of God, nor promote the word of God, is not doing the work of God. Therefore, any religion that sanctions the killing and eating of God's creatures is not doing the work of God. As a result, they often find themselves needing the cop-out phrase "The Lord works in mysterious ways," because it is the dogma of that religion which works in mysterious ways, not God. The religions want you to follow their ways, yet if something doesn't make sense to your instinct or your intellect, they resort to the cop-out, which plays on the frailties of human emotion. Then, religion introduces the element of fear to coerce you into following their misguided ways. To ensure *their* future, they instill a belief in you that if you don't follow this religion, God will punish you. They make you think that God is about fear, but in truth only meat-eating religion is about fear. God is about love. Sadly, people have followed this nonsense out of fear of God, so they live their life by creating fear, perpetuating fear and murdering innocent animals (more fear). Others follow this primrose path out of their innate need for spirituality, even if it violates their instincts. To move toward God we need to move away from evil, fear-creating lifestyles and blind faith in religions, and toward truth and love, which are godly attributes and behavior. Those who proudly proclaim to be God-fearing Christians should understand that God is not to be feared. God is love. Only in the realm of meat-eating religion is there this fear that they create for others and live by for themselves. Why be fearful? Simply live a life of truth and love and you can bask in its glow.

Moreover, even if there was a realm of punishment wrought by a loving God, it would be to punish evil actions, e.g. killing the innocent, not the pursuit of truth and love. In no uncertain terms, punishment and fear are tools of sociopaths, not of God.

In truth, God does not work in mysterious ways. God and his precepts are very plain to see if you are just willing to step outside The Big, Evil Lie to see them. And any religion whose intention is to really do the work of God must do the same thing.

> *"I care not much for a man's religion if his dog and cat are not the better for it."*   – Abraham Lincoln

Peace, truth, love, harmony for all, and even God, exist only collectively, and exclusively, and without hypocrisy, in a vegan world. If you want to feel God, if you want to see God, if you want to know God, then walk in God's path. It is a vegan path.

Original Sin

Christianity is the predominant religion on the planet and is faced with having to offer the masses some explanation as to why things are the way they are. "God works in mysterious ways" sometimes just doesn't cut it. Ergo, Christianity criminalizes sex as the dirty deed from which all others emanate. They will attempt to make you believe that you were "born of your mother's sin," and hope that you are shaken up enough to repeat this to your children, and them to their children. And so the real problem continues to grow and mutate through the ages.

In Genesis 1:27 God created Adam and Eve, and then immediately said unto them: "Be fruitful and multiply." So how is this a sin, exactly? Firstly, the answer lies in the fact that religion needs to criminalize something other than that which keeps them in business – meat. Secondly, they need to instill a disempowering, fear-creating, convoluted philosophy over which you have no control, and then threaten your eternity if you even question this nonsense in the first place.

The "sins of the flesh" have nothing to do with sex, but they are, rather, simply the sins of the flesh – as in eating it.

An interesting aside to this is the understanding of the word "sin." According to *Webster's New World Dictionary*, the word sin means "the breaking of religious law." Right there in the dictionary, religion has succeeded in making this a criminal act. And, where there is a criminal act, punishment is sure to follow, so you'd better be fearful. However, the word sin in ancient Hebrew, "chet," actually means "to miss the mark." Even if sex was somehow a sin, Christianity criminalizes it, whereas the true meaning of the word really implies to do better next time. In reality, the concept of "sin" is not to automatically create powerless victims, rather, it is to give you self-empowerment. To pursue excellence is the real essence of "sin." A running back on a football team commits a sin if he gets tackled while carrying the ball. He commits an even larger sin if he refuses to get up. The running back overcomes sin when he gets up, brushes himself off, gets back in formation and runs again, this time just a little bit harder.

The word sin has been corrupted by Christianity to instill a fear of something that God actually told us to do (and God didn't even mention marriage at that point). Christianity developed a smoke screen to the real problem and, in doing so, removed your individual sovereignty and your empowerment to make things better. That itself is truly a sin, using any definition you like.

Your mother's "original sin" was not to give you life, but rather to take the life of a chicken, call it nuggets and then offer it to you as food. Call it original sin, weakness of the flesh or anything else for that matter, but it is little more than the first time each of us swallows the flesh of a murdered animal.

The intent and scope of this book is not to disparage religion, per se. However, the purpose of this book is most definitely to get you to your divine power, and fulfill the original promise to lay before you the road map to paradise. Truth is an obligation and a responsibility, as well as a privilege and an honor. If any religion presents blockages toward this goal then we must step back, acknowledge it, and correct our path to get to that goal. Remember that religion is about religion, whereas God is God. The perceived connection between the two is a millennial and problematic relationship, and little more.

Hell On Earth

Hell is often thought of as a place where existence is continually dreadful and painful. Hell and evil go hand-in-hand. Ironically, religions that condone eating meat use hell as a weapon of fear to keep people faithfully blind, yet it is this practice that helps to create such dreadful conditions in the first place. It is also the very essence of a self-fulfilling prophecy.

Meat is dreadful and painful to those whose bodies are looked upon as food. Further, meat is no less dreadful and painful to those who preach love and compassion out of one side of their mouths while consuming this meat with the other. Fear, confusion, hypocrisy and disease plague all who reside on a planet engaged in the hellish lifestyle of meat.

In the name of God, though actually just a misguided belief in God through religion, many people live their lives opposed to the true values of God. This is hell. Pursue truth, embrace the true values of God, and hell may very well vanish, and, not coincidentally, so too would many religions.

Think of hell as any place where there is suffering. Meat is suffering. It is impossible for any religion that condones meat to get you to utopia, paradise or heaven. They don't even truly or accurately represent it. Meat is suffering and does not (and cannot) bring about paradise any more than does a suicide bomber. Meatism, and religion that condones meatism, explicitly create hell on Earth. If you want to get to paradise, you must not participate in meat-eating religion. If you want to get to paradise, you must embrace God. Paradise is the place where God lives. Veganism and its principles offer us the only highway to paradise and the direct connection to God.

Chapter 12

God

If you had been born without an olfactory system you could not understand the smell of freshly cut grass. Someone could try to explain it to you, but the very concept of smell, much less the actual aroma of cut grass, would be impossible to grasp. If you were born blind, you could not possibly fathom "blue." But the color would still exist.

We know things exist that we can't see, hear, taste, touch or smell, such as love or a dolphin's sonar. Unfortunately, there are also things that exist that even those of us with our five senses intact do not experience because of a self-imposed "blindness."

Meat-eating mankind pursuing God is very much like someone looking at a picture on the wall and then closing his eyes. He still has the necessary equipment in order to see the picture, but has chosen to shut himself off from it. But the picture still exists. What we do and how we live can offer greater "sight" or darker blindness. Meat eaters have the necessary equipment to "see" God, it's just been veiled.

It is critically important to begin a chapter on God with this understanding: there are powers and an existence that, for whatever reasons (lifestyle and choice amongst them), we perhaps cannot "see." This discussion will not anthropomorphize God, that is, attribute human characteristics to Him. Only misguided religion does that. Trying to describe the smell of cut grass to someone born without an olfactory nerve would only serve to distort the true scent, since this person would have no point of reference. So let's keep it simple.

Faith No More

Faith is largely a belief in something that cannot be seen. A society that engages in a lifestyle that is antithetical to God cannot see God. Trying to experience God while participating in murder (of people or animals) is like trying to see a painting with eyes clouded by cataracts. The tool you need is damaged. But the tool we need to see God is, fortunately, deep within each of us. If you become vegan, it would be hard for you not to become more loving, truthful, humane, happier, healthier and, therefore, more enlightened. As society becomes vegan, the painting on the wall that had been fuzzy and abstract becomes clear. But it was always there.

If you want to embrace God, why pursue faith? Faith is a tool of those who cannot embrace God. If you want to begin a direct connection to God, you simply must behave accordingly. You can think of spirituality as a "love connection," because spirituality is the connectedness of all souls. And remember, the essence of souls is love. So what spirituality is there, can there really be, in a murdering environment? If you want to connect to God, to all love, you must shun concepts of faith (blindness) and pursue and engage in the appropriate and necessary behavior (proper love) to your desired destination (enlightenment and God).

No matter how we live our lives, love is still love, truth is still truth, paradise is still paradise and God is still God, but because of our brutal, meat-eating ways, we can have none of it.

Keep It Simple

The universe exists. Simple. Some power, force or energy created it. Also simple. You can call this power God, Nature,

Buddha, The Divine or anything else, for that matter, but the very fact of our being here proves such a power exists. Religions attempt to personify this power, knowing full-well that meat eaters, with their many blockages, cannot see it. So they have given themselves license to dress Him in beards and robes. This personification helps keep the faithful blind in their belief, or drive away those who sense spirituality but reject the fairytale.

Scientists turned off by the fairytale try to dispel God entirely, citing the Big Bang theory of a large, isolated cosmic explosion that created the universe. Even if the Big Bang theory is accurate, does this mean God doesn't exist? If a bomb explodes, didn't someone build it?

Why attempt to personify this power beyond simply the acknowledgement and recognition of it? Any attempt at personification will only serve to distort it. The words we use to describe this power are a vain attempt at understanding something that isn't understandable with human words – certainly not a human language that contains "meat." Faith is not the answer, it is only more of the problem.

> *"By love he may be gotten and holden, but by thought or understanding, never."* – The Cloud of Unknowing

Sight Without Eyes

Sometimes people talk about an afterlife in which they will be reunited with lost loved ones. If such a place exists, you won't "see" your loved ones, as you won't have eyes. Though it can seem perhaps somewhat esoteric and abstract, the reality is the human body, the human condition, and its senses and its choices are actually the limiting factors to what we "see." When we're physically alive, we have two eyeballs that look straight ahead, and the rest of our body (including our eyelids) operates as blinders. In this spiritual realm, "vision" is complete and total and far beyond the capabilities of our five senses. This is enlightenment.

Enlightenment offers vision in the absence of eyeballs and can be described as many things. There are a lot of thoughts, senses and emotions for which there simply are no words. Even one language has words that have nuances and subtleties that another language doesn't. Capisce? One of the ways enlightenment can be attained is via "pure thought." Pure thought is the realm that exists in each of us which hardly any of us actually use. Most people think only using data that has been obtained by their five senses. But pure thought is a higher, accessible function of the brain that allows for greater knowledge.

> *"Few are those who see with their own eyes and feel with their own hearts."* — Albert Einstein

Accepting the scientists' theory of the Big Bang, the Judeo-Christian theory of Adam and Eve, or other cosmic or mystical theories is like trying to understand blue without eyeballs. There are, however, universal concepts that describe aspects of this power that we all can grasp. Truth, love and enlightenment are some of the concepts that can give you a glimpse into the universal power. Unfortunately, in the case of meat eaters, these concepts exist only to a point. Love exists only within a very small circle, sometimes referred to as "family." But aren't we all family?

As with a plumbing blockage, if water isn't getting to the faucet it doesn't mean water doesn't exist. Meat eaters have blockages of the heart, blockages of the mind and blockages of the soul. God exists, but if you have such a blockage in the path of love you will not, and cannot, see God, for God is love. Killing and eating God's animals creates monumental blockages. If God is love, then love is God. If X equals Y, then Y equals X. It is no more complex than simple mathematics. Where love exists, God exists – they are the same. Where love does not exist completely, without blockages, God is like a dry faucet, no matter how thirsty you may be.

The Common Thread

Virtually all beliefs in God, or belief in no God for that matter, have a commonality that nearly serves to prove the existence of this force. Whether you are atheist, agnostic, existentialist, Jewish, Christian, Hindu, Buddhist, Naturalist, Muslim or otherwise, God is the same. (Yes, even for the atheist.)

> *"I cannot say, 'That chair is not there,' if there is no chair there to say it about."*   – Madeleine L'Engle

Atheism is a rejection of all beliefs of religion and, therefore, of God. Atheists see religion as meritless, and then conclude that if religion holds no value, there must not be a God. However, God and religion have nothing to do with one another. There are probably a few atheists out there who simply disbelieve any existence beyond that which they can smell, taste, touch, hear or see. But blindness is sometimes more than faulty equipment, it is a foolish choice. To them, I suppose, bombs exist but nobody built them. But existence is existence despite the worst of religion. It is religion's inept anthropomorphism of God's existence that is fatally flawed. God's existence is downright instinctual, and even the practice of atheism struggles with this. If it didn't, "atheism" wouldn't even be a word, it would just be "nothing-ism." Atheists' vehement denial of God is in some ironic ways almost actual evidence that He exists (or that they instinctually believe He exists).

While atheists believe in the spontaneous appearance of bombs, agnostics reason that a human mind simply cannot understand the realm beyond the physical, so they attempt to live their lives without denying or embracing God. This is a lifelong attempt at walking on a very narrow balance beam that has nothing propping it up. It is like refusing to believe (or disbelieve) that the word processing software in your computer exists simply because when you take your computer apart you cannot see it or understand how it works. The mere fact that you are typing a letter should indicate that it, quite patently, exists, whether you understand it or not.

The computer analogy can also serve to further illustrate pure thought. Today's PCs require their own software in order to function. However, there is a much more powerful system lurking on the horizon. With the advent of the Internet, virtually all computers can be connected, so it is no longer necessary for each individual PC to have word processing or any other type of software physically loaded onto it. There are systems being developed that will allow your PC to access whatever software or information it needs from the World Wide Web at any time. The software-laden computers we know today will eventually be replaced by faster, streamlined terminals that we would use to access any and all software we need. This would be a far more advanced system. In some ways the difference between these two computer systems is very much like the difference between our brains and pure thought.

Actually, the difference between these two computer systems is important for many reasons, but there is one relevant factor here in discussing agnosticism. While agnostics hold that the physical brain cannot grasp a nonphysical realm, they overlook that a greater knowledge than the brain is already in existence. Similar to a streamlined terminal that can function in any capacity when it accesses a centralized database but is limited in its capabilities in isolation, our brains have the ability to use not just data obtained by the physical senses, but to access a "database" of infinite information. In very simplistic terms, this is pure thought, which is, or should be, a natural function of the brain.

> *"Information is not knowledge."*   – Albert Einstein

Pure thought allows the brain to think and is the commonality of all brains. But the usage of pure thought exists in the realm, and only in the realm, of pure love, the commonality of all souls. It is the source of all knowledge, whereas the brain is usually only used for the storage of data obtained by the physical senses. The human brain cannot fully understand God when used in this way, but this doesn't mean He doesn't exist. Firstly, one does not have to fully understand God to know God, just as you don't have to fully understand your spouse to know him or her. Secondly, and more to the point, the inability to understand God also has to do with veils created by vicious, ungodlike lifestyles – meat. Earlier we learned that there is actually a loss of brain function in feral children caused by their isolation from human society. This is no different. The isolation from God caused by eating meat causes us to lose the ability to access the pure thought our brains are capable of.

Nonetheless, there is a source of all knowledge and all power (and all love) that exists outside of us and our brains, or better put, irrespective of us and our brains, whether we know it or not, whether we use it or not. Pure thought can be accessed via the brain, and then the brain can store those lessons learned. But this is not how our meat-eating society is structured because pure thought does not exist in meatism. Pure thought is part and parcel of proper love. In meatism, the physical brain and pure thought are disconnected.

If you go to school and you learn that Christopher Columbus set sail on the Niña, the Pinta and the Santa Maria, you simply store that as data in your brain. You did not *think* that information. Even when you learn the multiplication table, what real thinking is involved? A huge problem with our education systems is that they are not teaching us to think, but to simply store data (and then serve hamburgers for lunch). So it is no surprise that we are a society that knows how to store data (most of it incorrect), but doesn't ever really think. What's worse, this "education" actually causes loss of brain function. Pure thought is interwoven with proper love, and they are the connection to God. Our meat-serving education systems are not really providing an education at all. They are like a large software store. They strive to install data (their data) in your brain while actually removing your ability to think.

Agnosticism can be aptly thought of as a software-based computer. This computer analogy should elucidate a higher order even if you don't understand the higher order itself. A readjustment of the tools we already use, or have at our disposal to use, such as the basics of truth and love, can yield this far greater order.

Then there are some people who look upon Nature as a force or power. These people don't spend energy denying or walking a tightrope of what may or may not be. They readily acknowledge a power, but they need to see it in a physical manifestation – Mother Nature.

Next to mention, though not in any particular order of significance, are the Eastern religions, such as Buddhism, that look inward to find God. They teach that the ultimate power, God, exists in the self. Through practices such as meditation, adherents believe they can reach this power, then they ask the question, if this power already exists in each of us, why do we need to "reach" it? It is an irony that they acknowledge and embrace, and they use it to dig deeper.

There are many, many religions in the world (and if you read the previous chapter you should understand why) and, thus, many ways of personifying God. The last I will mention here is the Judeo-Christian perspective. This entails looking outside the self to a heavenly realm to find an external God.

Are you beginning to see a common thread? If not, let me help you. Religion means nothing. Existence means everything. We all agree that "good," "just," "enlightened" and "love" are universal elements to our existence, or to what we would like for our existence. (Meat eaters, however, live every day of their lives in direct contrast to these elements.) At their core, these four words mean the same thing, so let's use just one of them – love. Love is what connects us all. Without it, we are a broken whole. With it, we are a connected oneness. In this connected realm, does God exist? Does it matter?

Love and God connect us all. How can we eat others? It is literally like killing and eating God.

There are some people who say that if there is no God then we can all be unscrupulous and mean. Certainly, in this case we would live in an ungodly world. Folks, if there is no God, if we are spinning off into space all alone, then that is more reason to love one another and to care for one another, not less. If we behaved in a loving manner toward all, we would live in a Godly world whether or not there is a God.

If the Judeo-Christian vision of an external God is correct, and that God told mankind we were created in His image, that would imply we contain His essence. If so, then the Buddhist vision of an internal God also exists. And if the Buddhist vision of God exists in the self, and there is a universal sameness of each self, then there must be an external God connecting each self. It is the same God. It is only religion that paints beards, fat bellies, robes and other adornments that distorts the picture. It is meat, an ungodly way of life, that has allowed religion to flourish and thus paint the distorted, graven images, taking you (intentionally or otherwise) away from love and God.

It is veganism, a lifestyle of proper love, which allows God to become omnipresent. Just imagine the absurdity of having love and God omnipresent and then somebody coming up to you trying to sell you on his religion. Perhaps he'd offer to buy you a steak dinner over which you could discuss it. He wouldn't need "ass" written across his chest, you'd see him for what he is from a mile away. Do you still feel that you need to see God with a beard?

Today, many religions look forward to the "Messianic Age," when the Earth will once again become paradise. One of the many reasons even flesh eaters enjoy believing in God, even if they can't see Him, is they feel God is just and fair, and in this Messianic era justice and fairness will prevail. Typically, this is a selfish desire, because these flesh eaters, being sociopaths, refuse to acknowledge that it is *their* way of life that is the unjust and unfair way that needs to be corrected. They only feel their own pain and think God will come and make everything just and fair *for them*. It simply doesn't work that way.

And The Wolf Shall Dwell With The Lamb

Most people believe in some form of Messiah. Whether in truth or lore, it makes no difference, the Messianic Age is thought of as a paradise. It is impossible for any paradise to exist – physical, mystical or otherwise – while the fear and pain of any creature, let alone ten billion a year, is being exploited in any way (much less for profit, selfishness and gluttony).

"And the wolf shall dwell with the lamb" is often used as the symbol of the Messianic Age. What is this if not a succinct portrait and essential requisite of the very nature of a paradise – veganism for all mankind and, in turn, all animalkind?

Whether the concept of the Messianic Age is fact or fantasy, veganism is to utopia as meatism is to dystopia. The answers to many of the world's problems come into perfect clarity from this vantage point. The farther we move from the basic principles of God, the more difficulties we will face, and the more we will cling to religion and its contradictory, self-sabotaging ideas of the Messiah.

The Choice Is Yours

One of the greatest gifts we humans have been blessed with is choice. The choice to do good or evil is entirely within the individual, as it should be, as this is the basis of individual sovereignty and free will. Unfortunately, many of those blessed with this free will who believe in God and a Messiah exercise their free will by doing all the things that are diametrically opposed to that God and the behavior necessary for that Messianic Age. It is very troubling that so many people pray to God because He is all-loving, yet refuse to give that love, in turn, to God's other creatures.

> *"In seeking to escape pain ourselves, why should we inflict it upon others?"*
> — The Buddha

We Are The World

The Messiah is here on Earth right now. The Messiah is you and the Messiah is me. In fact, we are all, or better put, can all be, the Messiah. The Messianic Age isn't created by faith or theory. It is created by behavior. Eating a hot dog while waiting for the Messiah is an absurdity, a hypocrisy and an outright impossibility. Eating meat is the very thing that needs to be expunged from the Earth to clear the way for such a Messianic Age.

Ask yourself what it means that God created man in His image. God doesn't have a physical appearance, so it cannot mean we were made to look like God. What it means is that God resides in each of us through love and, just as God has the power to create, so do we. We can create paradise or we can create ... what we've created. It is an amazing power, and an even more amazing responsibility. Each of us must take responsibility for our own actions, and behave as we would want God to behave. Clearly, our choices thus far have created the dystopian world in which we currently live. We can choose another path, but it's entirely up to you and me to create the type of world in which we want to live.

"I shall tell you a great secret, my friend. Do not wait for the final judgment, it takes place every day."
– Albert Camus

We all like to think that God is just. We take comfort in thinking that no matter what bad things may happen to us, there will be a final judgment and a final justice. But remember, we were created in the image of God. Rather than hoping that all wrongs done to you will be ultimately righted, you should right all the wrongs you do to others – you have that power. Pursue truth, pure thought and proper love, as this is where God lives. He actually never moved. We did.

To move away from a dystopia and toward our utopian potential, sovereignty of the individual must be cherished and respected. This sovereignty belongs with all the Earth's inhabitants, not just some. When we all respect the sovereignty of each and every individual, we can no longer exploit or kill them. To stop the dystopia and begin the utopia we must all be vegan, and we all must live by justice for others, not just for ourselves. This behavior is mandated in a Messianic Age.

People also like the notion of a strong God, so that He can protect us. Again, we were created in God's image. Mustn't we protect all others who can't protect themselves? That is the correct usage of individual sovereignty, to help others. It reinforces and ensures continuing individual sovereignty, even our own.

The Messianic Age can be upon us the instant we all realize the Messianic Age can be upon us. All we each need to do is behave in accordance with the paradigm of such an age. Eating animals and the Messianic Age are mutually exclusive. God has already bestowed upon us the ability to have a utopia, yet sitting around waiting for Him to force it upon us while we use our lives to create dystopia is pretty much the seed of all evil, not to mention a huge farce.

God is not evil. God is not farcical. God is truth. God is love. God just is. This is demonstrated by us all, human and nonhuman animal, sharing a distinct common characteristic that we would not have were we created randomly. That is, we are all driven to and by love.

Every corporation has a board of directors that convenes in a room aptly called a boardroom. Similarly, God convenes in the realm of love and truth aptly called paradise. Paradise, by its nature, cannot contain meat or those who partake of meat. Meat is the antithesis of love and truth. Meat is the antithesis of paradise. Meat eaters are the very thing that the Earth needs to purge in order to enter into a Messianic era. If you want to realize paradise and God, you must be vegan.

Some people ask, "What's the point of me becoming vegan? There will still be billions of cows and pigs and sheep and chickens slaughtered even if I stop eating them. It makes no difference." It makes a huge difference to each one of God's creatures that doesn't end up on your plate and is, in fact, the difference between good and evil. Creating a true paradise requires all people to participate, but the improbability of such an event taking place should not hinder you from doing your part immediately. One by one, until we are one.

Chapter 13

The Good Book

Whether you believe in the Bible or not, it is certainly fair to say that the Bible has laid the foundation of Western society. Whether the Bible is literal truth, metaphorical truth or just interesting folklore really doesn't matter. It holds inherent value either way, which makes it even more powerful. So, within the framework of a Judeo-Christian society, a proper and just perspective on veganism cannot be complete without pointing out that the Bible tells us to be vegan.

Setting The Record Straight

Whether you interpret the Sixth Commandment as "Thou shalt not kill" or "Thou shalt not murder," it can offer tremendous insight to those seeking it. Unfortunately, this has become a slogan that religions use for their own purposes, which often have nothing whatsoever to do with the phrase's real meaning. "Thou shalt not murder" means, I think, thou shalt not murder. It doesn't mean thou shalt not murder just me. God is speaking of all his creations "wherein there is a living soul." Some people say this commandment applies only to our behavior toward other humans. Where, oh, where does it say that? This is simple denial necessary to the meat eater's Big Lie.

Some people like to say that murder and killing are different. They suggest that if you make a person dead you have murdered, but if you make an animal dead you have killed. How convenient. Firstly, when God refers to the world and his creations as "good," there has yet to be murder (meat), or even killing. This is known as the Garden of Eden – paradise. Secondly, taking the life of innocent, nonaggressive, sentient beings that would have, but for our action, every interest in continuing to live is murder. Thirdly, do you really think the solution to creating paradise lies in a debate over the difference between murder and killing? To be clear, there may very well be a fatal act that does not rise to the level of murder, but systematically killing animals and devouring their dead bodies cannot possibly come under the heading of self-defense or euthanasia. The Big Lie facilitates a hope that eating animals is a loophole in God's law, whereas in reality it abates truth and love, causes injury and harm and is, therefore, evil and anti-God.

"Love thy neighbor" is another well-known Biblical phrase which simply means to love thy neighbor, not just if thy neighbor happens to be 5 feet 7 inches, 117 pounds and 36-24-36. In fact, our neighbors are not only human females (or males) with perfect figures, but also cows, rabbits, chickens, deer, mice, pigs and, depending upon where you live, maybe even elephants and giraffes. If you feel uncomfortable around lions or alligators, simply don't take up residency in a place where they will be your neighbors. But if you did, in fact, love thy neighbor, you would probably not feel uncomfortable around any of God's creatures. There is no hypocrisy in the realm of truth or in the presence of proper love and God.

"The meek shall inherit the Earth" offers even more insight. Meek means gentle and mild, not aggressive and combative. One who is meek is vegan. Murder (or killing) is the essence of aggression and is the opposite of meek.

The Messianic Age is often referred to as the time when the meek shall inherit the Earth and "the wolf shall dwell with the lamb." Are you starting to see a common denominator to it all? That common denominator is a vegan way of life. Planet Utopia can only be vegan.

The Forbidden Fruit is ... Flesh

In Jewish and Christian beliefs the Garden of Eden was paradise. One day, something happened that changed paradise forever. We've all heard of the forbidden fruit and believe that paradise changed when Eve ate this "fruit." Many people think this forbidden fruit was an apple or a fig. But why would God be upset that man (and woman) ate an apple or a fig? You don't know why? Of course you don't know why, because God would not be upset that man ate apples and figs. In fact, God gave us these as food for us to eat: "I have given you every herb yielding seed ... and every tree, in which is the fruit of a tree yielding seed ... to you it shall be for food" (Genesis 1:29). This sentence is as clear as any sentence can be; apples and figs, or any fruit for that matter, have not been forbidden by God.

In reality, the forbidden fruit was not a fruit at all. It is simply a symbolic term. But we must get past the symbolism to understand the true meaning of that from which we were to abstain.

The forbidden fruit was flesh.

Flesh is the very thing that instantly destroys paradise. The Garden of Eden was a paradise. The Garden of Eden was one hundred percent vegan. A true paradise must logically be vegan. When the very concept of flesh came into existence, paradise was destroyed. When the hunt began, paradise was obliterated. *You* cannot have paradise if *I* don't have paradise. *We* cannot have paradise if *they* do not have paradise; it is an absolute impossibility. We are all connected, as we are all the physical embodiment of the spirit of God. We cannot bring fear and murder to one of God's creatures without destroying paradise for ourselves. In paradise, every body that houses the spirit of God (including animals) must live in peace and harmony.

> *"Cruelty to animals is as if humans did not love God."*
> – Cardinal Newman

Paradise was not blown up by a bomb, it was eaten away by our teeth. In fact, bombs are not even close to our root problem. Meat is violence. Meat is the very antithesis of all that is good, just, enlightened and loving. Meat is the very debasement of paradise. Meat is the cornerstone of dystopia. Apples and figs are food. Meat is both the root problem and the forbidden fruit.

To want paradise yet refuse this first truth means to start the insidious process all over again. Five thousand years ago God said, "Thou shalt not kill." Yet today, the meat and dairy industries need you to believe something very different. What, or whom, will you believe, God and love or meat and dairy?

If you choose paradise over dystopia, proper love over raw emotion, truth over deceit, humanity over cruelty, and God over godless, then you must follow the mandate set down by that God on how to live in His "good" world. And, just in case 6.5 billion times is not enough, "herb-yielding seed ... and every tree ... to you it shall be for food."

Urgent Advisory

It is important to note that only at the very beginning of the Bible, where we can actually see a paradise, does God refer to the world as "good." Once the forbidden flesh was consumed, the world becomes a violent dystopia. Therefore, to cite a passage from anywhere but the beginning of the Bible (when things were good) as justification for some type of behavior only furthers violent and dystopian behavior. In fact, most of the Bible is a case study in how *not* to behave. Yet, the faithfully blind recite it as justification. Justification of what? More violence? The only passages that should serve as a case study in how we are to behave to create paradise and sustain peace are from the beginning of the Bible, when the world, and our existence, was good and at peace. From this vantage point, it will be easy to see how and why peace changed to violence, and how we can change it back. As always, to best understand something you need to step back to the beginning. You need to understand the genesis.

> *Genesis 1:24-25*
> *"And God said: 'Let the Earth bring forth the living creature after its kind, cattle, and creeping thing, and beast of the Earth after its kind.' And it was so. And God made the beast of the Earth after its kind, and the cattle after their kind, and every thing that creepeth upon the ground after its kind; and God saw that it was good."*

Here is the simple evidence for all to see that at the beginning of Creation God sees things as good. It is only after man begins eating meat that God no longer refers to *anything* as good.

> *Genesis 1:26-28*
> *"And God said: 'Let us make man in our image, after our likeness; and let them have dominion over the fish of the sea, and over the fowl of the air, and over the cattle, and over all the Earth, and over every creeping thing that creepeth upon the Earth.' And God created man in His own image, in the image of God created He him; male and female created He them. And God blessed them; and God said unto them: 'Be fruitful, and multiply, and replenish the Earth, and subdue it; and have dominion over the fish of the sea, and over the*

fowl of the air, and over every living thing that creepeth upon the Earth.'"

"Dominion" is a responsibility to care for others, not a license to molest or kill them. The next time you hire a babysitter, understand that you are allowing her to have dominion over your children. You should use your dominionship over others as you would like your babysitter to use hers. This passage clearly states that we were created in God's image to do God's work. Man was given the job of ultimate caretaker and, instead of doing his job properly, he has become the ultimate killing machine (and then goes to church to pray for God's mercy and compassion for *himself* and *his* family).

> *"I cannot think it extravagant to imagine that mankind are no less, in proportion, accountable for the ill-use of their dominion over the lower ranks of beings than for the exercise of tyranny over their own species. The more entirely the inferior creation is submitted to our power, the more accountable we must seem for the mismanagement of it."*   – Alexander Pope

It is our first job to care for all of God's creatures. Service to others is the very meaning of life. A world full of flesh-eating people who look to God to solve problems is the essence of a police state. Rather than living up to their own responsibilities, as individual sovereigns, they live any way they want, and then look to God for justice. A police state, by man or God, is about control over others – far and away from peace, harmony and God.

Genesis 1:29-31
"And God said: 'Behold, I have given you every herb yielding seed, which is upon the face of all the Earth, and every tree, in which is the fruit of a tree yielding seed; to you it shall be for food; and to every beast of the Earth, and to every fowl of the air, and to every thing

that creepeth upon the Earth, wherein there is a living soul, I have given every green herb for food.' And it was so. And God saw every thing that He had made, and, behold, it was very good. And there was evening and there was morning, the sixth day."

The first sentence of this passage tells us unequivocally that *plants* are our food. Once again, apples and figs are plants. Therefore, it wasn't an apple or a fig that Eve ate which upset God. Let us finally, once and for all, lay that ridiculous notion to rest.

This same passage goes on to state that these plant foods are food for all of us – human and nonhuman animal – "Every thing that creepeth upon the Earth … I have given every green herb for food." In fact, it was only after man began eating meat that animals also started eating meat (once a paradise changes, all of its parts also change). The supposed food chain to which meat eaters refer to justify their habits is nothing more than their own dystopian creation. Then, once created, they point to it to justify The Big Lie.

And, oh yes, this passage makes a very clear distinction between plants, which are food, and animals, which have souls. It clearly states that *all* animals have a soul. And God saw this as "very good." Then our meat-eating habits needed this to be untrue, so we needed to change truth. However, truth does not change, we just die of cancer and heart disease.

The forbidden fruit was one of God's creatures, which we were put on Earth to care for, and which we actually killed and consumed. There is nothing more grotesque. Subsequently, God's "good" paradise was destroyed. *Never again* does God refer to anything as "good."

Genesis 3:1-3
"And he (the serpent) said unto the woman: 'Yea, hath God said Ye shall not eat of any tree of the garden?' And

> *the woman said unto the serpent: 'Of the fruit of the*
> *trees of the garden we may eat; but of the fruit of the*
> *tree which is in the midst of the garden, God hath said:*
> *Ye shall not eat of it, neither shall ye touch it, lest ye*
> *die.'"*

It is essential to understand the difference between "the fruit of the trees of the garden" and what is meant by "the tree in the midst of the garden." The former simply refers to the actual fruit, as in apples and figs. In the latter, the word "midst" means "central part." The central part of the Garden of Eden is God and his "fruit" (as in "be fruitful and multiply"). God's "fruit" is the human and nonhuman animals "wherein there is a living soul" (the soul being our common connection to God), which God prohibited Adam and Eve from eating. God also refers to the tree in the midst of the garden as the "tree of the knowledge of good and evil" (Genesis 2:17) and the "tree of life" (Genesis 3:22). What could be more evil than denying life to any of God's fruit?

Genesis 3:4-5
"And the serpent said unto the woman: 'Ye shall not
surely die; for God doth know that in the day ye eat
thereof, then your eyes shall be opened, and ye shall be
as God, knowing good and evil.'"

The last line is very telling – "... knowing good *and* evil." The "tree of the knowledge of good and evil" adds evil to our otherwise good dimension. Evil is added because eating of this tree (eating flesh) fundamentally destroys paradise. Paradise is destroyed when even just one constituent of that paradise is violated. You can choose to eat meat, but you cannot eat meat without creating evil.

Hypocrisy No More

Eating animals while praying to God for peace is the greatest absurdity and hypocrisy in all the universe. It's time we stopped praying to God for things we claim we want while doing everything to the contrary. If you want paradise, you must do your part. Flesh is forbidden in utopia not by force, but by the very nature of what is necessary to a utopia – peace, love, harmony and service to others; the essence of God and his favor. If you want paradise, you must be vegan.

The Return To Paradise

Logic and reason, supported by the written word of the Bible, backed by the very meaning and essence of humanity will, once and for all, elucidate the meat-eating world's forbidden truth: Meat is the destroyer of paradise. It is vile, unhealthy, evil, dystopian, anti-humane and anti-God, in no uncertain terms.

Albert Einstein said that nothing would benefit humankind more than the evolution to a vegetarian diet. If the Bible is nothing more than a story, Einstein's premise is one hundred percent accurate. However, if the Bible, or at least some portion of it, is an actual accounting of history, then Einstein's theory is still accurate, with one minor, technical exception. Veganism is not so much an evolution, but a return to what once was. In either case, Einstein's tenet is fundamentally correct. From the Bible's account, our planet was once a paradise. After all, it was a loving God who created it.

Have we come to the end of the story, or have we come full circle, or to a new beginning? Will *you* perpetuate evil or live a life of love and humanity (and health)?

As it should be, the choice is yours.

Chapter 14

Vivisection

Paradise is a place of truth and love, and the path to, or back to, paradise is clear. If you create another's suffering, or even close your eyes to another's suffering, paradise soon becomes greeting card material.

Whereas truth and love beget more truth and love, evil and death beget more evil and death. Eating animals is an evil and problematic behavior. Thanks to meat, paradise is gone, and all diseases and conditions that plague our godless, meat-eating world need a solution. Sociopathic and inept problem solving replaces veganism and truth in search of "solutions." This continues to take evil to new lows. The most evil of evils, the vilest act against God, the lowest of lows is known as vivisection.

Vivisection is experimentation performed on living animals. Oftentimes, these experiments are performed without anesthesia, and even with anesthesia, the aftereffects can be excruciatingly painful. The physical wounding usually leads to death, but in many cases it is the pain itself that is lethal. One of the more routine experiments is pouring corrosive materials into the eyes of an animal, which is so excruciating the animal will often kill itself by banging its head against the floor or breaking its own back from futile bodily gyrations in an attempt to get away from the pain.

"Vivisection, in my opinion, is the blackest of all crimes that man is at present committing against God and His fair creatures."   – Mahatma Gandhi

The propaganda of vivisection purports its use to be finding treatments for diseases plaguing man. But it is important to remember that these are diseases that plague meat-eating man. Meat eaters eventually acquire one or more of a variety of ailments from brutalizing animals and believe they need to brutalize more animals to find cures. Yet the hard reality is vivisection has yielded little in the way of cures for anything. Don't expect those engaged in the practice of vivisection, and who make huge amounts of money from it, to ever let you know the truth. They need you to believe something worthwhile comes from what they do, so the propaganda strives to convince you these are wholehearted Samaritans, sacrificing themselves in the pursuit of cures for terrible diseases. The truth is these are demented minds, albeit well-spoken and "educated," engaged in financial profiteering at the expense of humanity. The bottom line is these savages inflict lethal pain on innocent animals. Good does not come from evil. Curing a violent lifestyle cannot come from more violence, and curing inhumanity cannot come from more inhumanity. Nothing good, just or decent comes from vivisection – nothing. If we lived a purposeful life, if we knew God, would we be so afraid to die that we would be grasping at the poisonous straws vivisection purports to offer?

"I abhor vivisection with my whole soul. I detest the unpardonable slaughter of innocent life in the name of science and of humanity so-called, and all the scientific discoveries stained with innocent blood I count as of no consequence."   – Mahatma Gandhi

There is one thing that vivisection does do very well. It buys luxurious winter homes for those engaged in the sinister practice. There are millions of government and private dollars up for grabs to researchers wanting to bestow their evil ways upon helpless animals. Your tax dollars go to mad scientists who like to take baby kangaroos from their mothers to observe their need for mothering, cut limbs off one animal and attach them to another, and implant electrodes in the brains of dogs and cats so they can know what will happen if they decide to put electrodes in *your* brain. These are just for openers, parts of Vivisection 101 that are considered so basic they are performed in just about every medical facility in the world.

We now know why the government doesn't just take the hundreds of million of dollars they throw away on vivisection and, instead, use it to educate its citizens on how to be healthy through a vegan lifestyle. Both vivisectionists and many in government would be out of business. That's probably why the pictures of animals in laboratories that leak out from time to time are suppressed as quickly as possible. Most people would be utterly outraged at the brutality, and might actually insist vivisection be stopped. Seeing animals forced to live with their bodies literally cut open and their organs hanging out while alive and conscious would probably cause quite a stir.

But perhaps not. A major part of the reason why the masses allow vivisection to continue has its roots in sociopathy, selfishness and hypocrisy. Firstly, meat eaters by definition are sociopathic and selfish, eating what they want despite the cruelty. Meat eaters are also painfully aware that they will not die from old age but rather from diseases plaguing meat eaters. As a result, despite truth and humanity, they want to believe the propaganda of vivisection, that just maybe a cure for a disease can be found. Secondly, the masses eat meat, so how altruistic can they be? They may despise the cruelty being inflicted upon animals in laboratories, but somewhere in their conscience they know that they have the blood of many animals on their hands.

Therefore, they can't push their antivivisection points too far before their own hypocrisy shines through.

> *"It is easy to take a stand on a remote issue, but [one] reveals his true nature when the issue comes nearer home. To protest about bullfighting in Spain or the slaughter of baby seals in Canada while continuing to eat chickens that have spent their lives crammed into cages, or veal from calves that have been deprived of their mothers, their proper diet, and the freedom to lie down with their legs extended, is like denouncing apartheid in South Africa while asking your [white] neighbors not to sell their houses to blacks."*
>
> – Peter Singer

Hypocrisy doesn't allow truth to flourish on one side of the equation because that would mean truth would have to flourish on the other side as well. Despite the inhumanity, meat eaters want, and think they need, the vivisectionists, who play on those frailties. The masses don't draw a hard line in the sand against vivisection because vivisectionists say they are only doing it to help humanity move forward. But how can torture move humanity forward? Nothing in the realm of truth is more absurd.

What is medically true for a mouse or a dog is not necessarily true for a human. Even if it were, it is a violation of all laws of humanity to trespass on their individual sovereignty, much less torture them. Truth and humanity can supply us with the insights we really need. Vivisectionists need you to make the leap of faith that torturing a dog will somehow help man. Not coincidentally, the same vivisectionists downplay humane methods and tools, such as computer models, that can be used to clearly understand man. Aside from the fact that computer models can offer far greater insight than burning out the eyes of a rabbit, and aside from the fact that we can test substances at a cellular level without making a cat live in a cage with its brains hanging out, those engaged in vivisection profit at our expense and the expense of justice and humanity.

> *"I sit on a man's back choking him and making him carry me, and yet assure myself and others that I am sorry for him and wish to lighten his load by all means possible – except by getting off his back."*   – Leo Tolstoy

Fool Me Once, Shame On You; Fool Me Twice, Shame On Me

When a child doesn't do his homework and watches television all day instead and then asks his parents to help him, often what the child is seeking is a way out of his responsibilities rather than actual help with his studies. Similarly, when people seek the help of vivisectionists, or seek to benefit from the work of vivisectionists, they do so in order to avoid taking responsibility for the results of their own irresponsible lifestyles.

Vegans do not want or need the "help" of vivisection. Vivisection cannot help or cure a poor lifestyle anyway. Neither paradise nor health exists in a laboratory. In the case of a parent who does the child's homework, that parent is really only hurting the child, not helping him. Similarly, in the case of vivisection, those seeking the cop-out are only being hurt more. Caveat emptor: Let the buyer beware.

> *"Nothing cruel is useful or expedient."*   – Cicero

Mengele's Mirror

What good has come from vivisection? Throughout this book I write about love and how proper love is a behavior, not just a philosophy or emotion. Remember, the same is true of evil. Evil isn't a "thing," but a behavior. When one inflicts pain upon another, that behavior is evil. It is an even greater evil when it is systematic and heartless under the guise of humanity – the very lifeblood of vivisection. Simply no good can come from vivisection because, at its core, vivisection is evil, and good does not come from evil.

But let's imagine for a moment that vivisection was responsible for curing heart disease. Microscopically, this can appear beneficial, as a few components of the Earth have been helped, i.e. those who suffer from heart disease. But macroscopically, because heart disease comes about from an unnatural and destructive lifestyle, curing this disease will only lead to far greater corrections in nature's order of things. Heart disease will be replaced by something far more deadly in order to create a balance in nature, just as for every illness that is cured, another ten appear to take its place. The brute force of evil science cannot ever effectively combat the gentle, just truths of nature. That's just the way it is. In other words, concealing the effects of an unnatural lifestyle can encourage more unnatural ways of living, or it can create a belief that the unnatural way of living is not unnatural. In either case, it fosters greater unnatural living, which will cause greater and greater calamities.

"Isn't man an amazing animal? He kills wildlife – birds, kangaroos, deer, all kinds of cats, coyotes, beavers, groundhogs, mice, foxes and dingoes – by the million in order to protect his domestic animals and their feed. Then he kills domestic animals by the billion and eats them. This, in turn, kills man by the million, because eating all those animals leads to degenerative and fatal health conditions like heart disease, kidney disease and cancer. So then man tortures and kills millions more animals to look for cures for these diseases. Elsewhere, millions of other human beings are being killed by hunger and malnutrition because food they could eat is being used to fatten domestic animals. Meanwhile, some people are dying of sad laughter at the absurdity of

man, who kills so easily and so violently and, once a
year, sends out cards praying for 'Peace on Earth.'"
  – Peace On Earth, by C. David Coates
  (excerpted from *Old MacDonald's Factory Farm*)

Evil In The Name Of Science

Every once in a while mad scientists make the headlines for
taking the heart out of a baboon and transplanting it into a
human being. These well-spoken evil-doers show the nation
the patient after the transplant, but where are all the
cameras just a few weeks later, after this patient has died?
Instead of the public seeing the real truth, that the patient
died, they just see that this patient has been "saved."

Sadly, this patient had spent his life killing animals to
eat them, then had a diseased heart as a result of all this
"food." Then the doctors kill a completely innocent baboon
to steal his heart and put it in someone who is going to die in
a few days anyway. But the shrewd promoters of vivisection
only show you the few seconds after the transplant, and they
don't show you the $100,000 cars (invariably with leather
interiors) in which the doctors drive away from the hospital.

The truth is, despite vivisection, heart disease is killing
one million people every year in the United States alone.
Heart disease can only be cured (and prevented) by the
adoption of a healthy, natural vegan diet. How interesting it
is to consider that sparing the lives of the cows, pigs,
chickens, fish, etc., will spare our own lives, which, in turn,
spares the lives of the animals that would otherwise end up
in laboratories. Death begets death, whereas saving lives
begets more saved lives.

"There will never be any peace in the world so long as
we eat animals."   – Isaac Bashevis Singer

Profiles Of Dementia

Ask yourself what kind of person could inflict lethal pain on a gentle animal. These people look nice, talk nice and have nice offices with impressive looking plaques and nameplates. They drive nice cars and have nice homes. Vivisectionists go by fancy titles such as "doctor," "professor" and "scientist," but remember, just because someone goes to college, has an excellent vocabulary and a lot of money, doesn't mean they aren't evil.

> *"If you have men who will exclude any of God's creatures from the shelter of compassion and pity, you will have men who will deal likewise with their fellow men."*   – St. Francis of Assisi

Some argue that vivisectionists are more misguided than they are evil and that they actually believe they are doing good. But is the animal's suffering lessened because of such a debate? If you were being abused, would you feel better knowing that the perpetrator believed he was doing you a favor? Whether they are deliberately harming animals, doing so to get their demented jollies, or are just ignorant of the suffering they are causing, remember that evil is a *behavior*. Those engaged in evil behavior are evil whether they sport horns, white coats, expensive suits or otherwise. And please don't be naive enough to think they wouldn't experiment on you if you hadn't a larynx and a mouth to protest.

Is vivisection love? Is it truth? Is it humanity? Is it freedom? Can it co-exist with individual sovereignty? Can it possibly exist in a Godly paradise? Vivisection is the very worst of mankind; it is torture for the sake of torture. It is nothing but the folly of a very dysfunctional mind and people. It is the fast lane on a one-way expressway out of paradise.

Your life represents either the principles of paradise or it doesn't. We must stop enslaving and torturing God's creatures, and we must liberate all those whose freedom we are denying. The first, most significant, most profound and yet simplest method for eliminating vivisection is to become vegan. You will no longer want or need the dark promises of this pseudo science. Once vegan, you can live a life of truth, humanity and love without any hypocrisy. The paradise *you* want is the paradise *you* can create.

> *"Wisdom is knowing what to do next ... virtue is doing it."*
> — David Starr Jordan

Part Two

"When health is absent wisdom cannot reveal itself, art cannot become manifest, strength cannot be exerted, wealth is useless and reason is powerless."
– Herophilies, 300 B.C.

Chapter 15

Health Care

*"Better to put a strong fence around the top of the cliff
than an ambulance down in the valley."*

– Joseph Malins

Health care is one of the great issues of our time. Unfortunately, what is commonly referred to as health care actually has very little to do with health. The immense governmental issue of health care is really about financing disease. Currently, our system is structured in such a way that there is far more money to be made from disease than from health. This entire structure detonates paradise, and all of us affected scatter in all the wrong directions. Ergo, health care is, sadly, not a quest for health but rather a mission to partake of the subsequent riches of disease. It is lamentable that many people enjoy it this way, believing they can somehow profit from it. Most people call this health care. I call it disease care.

The Fallacious Cycle Of Health Care

The United States of America is a nation whose economy, to a large extent, revolves around animal products. We are a nation dying of diseases caused by eating meat. We are a nation embroiled in debating the issue of health care. We are a nation whose economy revolves around animal products.

Can you write the next line? The issue of health care has no beginning and no end in a meat-eating society, and those perpetuating the lamentable call this job security.

The problematic issue of health care is not going to be solved until such time as we simply want to solve it. In fact, an "issue" is just one of those unsolvable riddles that is often developed for the purpose of keeping those debating the issue busy. An issue has many sides to foster debate, but right and wrong have little to do with issues. Many politicians are prestigiously employed because of animal agriculture. Do these problem-solvers really want to solve the problems? They would be better off if they did. Unfortunately, they don't see it that way because the continual debate would no longer be in existence, and neither would their prestigious jobs in which they get to control other lives.

Most people live their lives, for all intents and purposes, begging for disease, then, once ill, want to be cured. Then the medical community rushes in, with sirens blaring, to profit from it all.

Eating meat causes fatigue and fosters our sedentary lifestyle in which we spend our leisure hours flopped in front of a TV. At dinnertime we prepare the seeds of disease care to feed our children. Feeding animal products to our children is not only cruelty to animals, it is one of the most gruesome forms of disease care, which is actually child abuse, ordaining that child's future to be replete with disease.

The High Cost (And Profits And Hypocrisy) Of Disease Care

People don't want to be ill, but most live their lives egging it on (no pun intended). The meat and dairy industries, and all those financially connected therewith, are only too happy to oblige and, as a result, the only thing growing faster than our waistlines and the cancers connected to animal products are the bank accounts connected to animal products. One of the more notable follies of this arrangement is McDonald's, whose marketing is especially geared toward children, and which also has a cancer charity for children called the Ronald McDonald House. At face value, this seems to be a humanitarian gesture by a company caring about its clientele. I have no doubt that many of those children, however, need the services of the Ronald McDonald House *because* of the marketing strategies and food served by McDonald's. I can't help suspect the Ronald McDonald House to be an intentional smoke screen. In any case, this is a very sad, disease-producing, confusion-causing scenario. Meat industries make money, McDonald's makes money, doctors make money and pharmaceutical companies make money. They all appear to be kindhearted Samaritans and, as a result, some politicians like to get in on the act, showing their support, all the while innocent children and animals are dying from the wares.

Take Two Of These (Forever), And Call Me In The Morning

Monitoring someone with elevated blood pressure does little but cost money, provide a large and regular income for the doctor, and practically ensure that, as time goes by, more drastic and more expensive measures will be needed. As with typical disease care, monitoring a patient for a couple of years almost invariably leads to prescribing "necessary" medications. These medications don't cure anything but rather conceal the ongoing internal destruction. Many pharmaceutical companies become enormously wealthy from this arrangement, and often offer doctors incentives to prescribe their products. After a few more years, surgery becomes necessary. This buys the surgeon his winter home in Florida. Politicians, meanwhile, whose salaries are paid by our taxes, debate the issue of health care, that is, how to finance all of this disease.

What's the result of all this? Firstly, consumers believing that going to the doctor, taking drugs and having surgery will bring about health is actually what keeps them in a state of disease and/or susceptible to disease. Secondly, this belief gives doctors a nice warm home in which to live in the winter. Thirdly, it provides huge profits for pharmaceutical companies, who promote and capitalize on patented chemical concoctions. (Interestingly, many of these patented drugs are often derived from the very same herbs that the medical community says are a waste of time in combating illness.) Fourthly, all of this health care maintains the need for continual debate over health care and how to finance it. This helps politicians accumulate wealth for themselves. Hey, c'mon now. The doctors need neighbors down Florida way.

Eating animals and animal products is the very foundation of disease and yet, because these products are the financial backbone of so many industries, few people will speak the truth. Most, as a result of The Big Lie, don't even know the truth. Heart disease, for example, is thriving in almost every man, woman and child who eats animal products, and it kills one million people every year in the United States alone. The enormous revenue generated by the animal product industries aside, the health costs involved are staggering. Just one heart bypass operation costs tens of thousands of dollars. The patient then needs lifelong, constant monitoring by a league of doctors and other health care professionals, pharmaceutical manufacturers, etc. And, yes, the patient usually needs a few more "procedures" along the way. And this is just one person.

After the animal product industries have been made wealthy, billions upon billions upon billions of dollars are thrown away on disease care, when true health care, care that truly fosters health, costs very little. Disease care is to health care as greed is to philanthropy, as brute force is to finesse, as killing is to humanity, as stupidity is to intelligence, and as meatism is to veganism.

Preventative Medicine

Much to their greedy chagrin, even those perpetuating this cycle know the costs associated with disease care are becoming too much to bear. As a result, slowly but surely, preventative medicine is becoming increasingly seen as a solution. But this preventative medicine means routine visits to your doctor so that he can monitor you even more and catch disease in its early stages. This still has nothing to do with preventing anything (other than preventing a reduction in doctors' incomes), nor with furthering health. This is simply better disease management. Conversely, true preventative medicine is not medicine at all, but simply another term for living the way nature intended.

> *"The doctor of the future will give no medicine, but will interest his patients in the care of the human frame, in diet and in the cause and prevention of disease."*
> – Thomas Edison

Do you suppose the medical and pharmaceutical industries might use Edison's quote as a slogan for their saturation advertising? Or do they do what they can to squelch such unprofitable statements?

Doctor, Doctor

Doctors (and politicians) are not the only culprits in the evil cycle of disease care. They have merely found a way to capitalize from it all. If you understand the power of the pyramids, you must take control over your life or somebody out there will do it for you, and it won't be to serve your best interests.

Changing the way the world eats is actually not the job of doctors. In most cases, they merely attempt to work with what they've got. In other words, when somebody who is ill comes into their offices they simply attempt to alleviate the illness at hand. Typically, this means alleviating the discomfort-causing symptoms. But this has nothing what-soever to do with solving the problem and making the patient healthy. The astounding fact is most doctors have practically no nutritional training. They learn chemistry and biology, but have little working knowledge of how what we ingest affects our well-being. They know how to prescribe drugs that mask the symptoms caused by unnatural eating and then, because drugs can't truly solve the problems caused by unnatural eating, they know how to cut out a tumor or an artery once it becomes clogged from that unnatural eating.

Since doctors have set themselves up as the source of information on health, they should be accountable for correct information. However, until doctors embrace the fact that it is living in accordance with nature that provides health, and not chemistry, "correct information" is really subjective poppycock. Further, while most doctors know there are many benefits to cutting out meat and dairy from the diet, as well as eating an abundance of fruits and vegetables, they still cannot see past their own early in-doctrination and The Big Lie. Plus, doctors have spent tens of thousands of dollars attending medical school and want their money's worth. Besides, even if they were to start espousing the truth, doctors could talk until they were blue in the face and many people simply would not listen. A good example of this is cigarettes. Even now that it is politically correct to oppose smoking and doctors are outspoken on its dangers, millions of people keep smoking.

> *"I think in the next ten or twenty years, we'll have evidence [showing that a vegetarian diet is superior] that is as strong as the evidence that cigarette smoking causes lung cancer. In my opinion, it's plenty strong enough now."* – T. Colin Campbell,
> Project Director of the China-Oxford-Cornell
> Diet and Health Project, the largest study of
> diet and health in medical history

Whereas "no smoking" is now politically correct, veganism is anything but politically correct, and most people won't heed the "V" word. There are some doctors who do go against conventional medicine by recommending a vegan diet, but they are scorned by their peers when they attempt to guide their patients against popular opinion. So sometimes doctors just tell their patients what they want to hear. After all, if the patients won't listen, the doctors might as well make money from it. This is, of course, no excuse, either for the doctors or the patients.

> *"Why must we be reticent about recommending a diet which we know is safe and healthy? We, as scientists, can no longer take the attitude that the public cannot benefit from information they are not ready for. I personally have great faith in the public. We must tell them that a diet of roots, stems, seeds, flowers, fruit and leaves is the healthiest diet and the only diet we can promote, endorse, and recommend."*
> – T. Colin Campbell,
> Project Director of the China-Oxford-Cornell
> Diet and Health Project

Much to the chagrin of the medical community at large, there are some doctors (unfortunately the smallest faction of all) who are proving that vegan diets are the *only* means to true health care. Dr. Dean Ornish, Dr. Michael Klaper, Dr. John McDougall, Dr. Julian Whitaker and Dr. Neal Barnard are some of the more notable who do promote health care in its most appropriate manner.

> *"The best doctors in the world are Doctor Diet, Doctor Quiet, and Doctor Merryman."*   – Jonathan Swift

Real Health Care

Neither doctors, pharmaceutical companies nor governments can create health from an unnatural lifestyle. One's own health is one's own responsibility, and being vegan, along with some form of exercise regimen, is the only true means of achieving effective health care. As the saying goes, you can pay now or pay later. Disease care can seem much less expensive, because you don't have to go out now and spend money on walking shoes or a gym membership, which don't seem imperative. Ironically, the far greater expense of a big-screen TV and recliner does not seem to bother most people. Consequently, after a few short, lazy years of being penny wise and dollar foolish lounging in front of their TVs, they are faced with more expenditure: doctors' visits, drugs and, eventually, surgeries, the costs of which are almost incalculable. The average meat-eating, disease-care-involved American is paying both now *and* later. The Big Lie helps to justify this and conceal the truth in their minds, so they simply blame the health care industry for their astronomical health care costs.

Not long ago I heard the famous talk show host Larry King reminisce about Jonas Salk, who developed the vaccine for polio. Larry King went on to tell the story of how Salk and his employees were all depressed after making their discovery because they had nothing left to do. Perhaps modern-day doctors have learned from Jonas Salk how to avoid depression. Contrary to disease care, teaching someone how and why they have elevated blood pressure and what they can do to bring it down costs very little money; hardly enough for a payment on a scooter, let alone a Mercedes. This is true health care, and it is based on philanthropy, finesse, intelligence and humanity.

"Your choice of diet can influence your long-term health prospects more than any other action you might take." – C. Everett Koop, former Surgeon General

Medications to control "monitored" conditions can cost hundreds of dollars every month. Since tax dollars are also at stake, true health care can save us a fortune, individually and collectively. The average American works until April every year just to pay his tax burden, and a substantial portion of this money fuels the counterproductive health care cycle. If this cycle, and the diseases that go with it, didn't need to be financed, you could have one heck of a vacation every year. Or just think how many veggie burgers and jogging shoes you could buy with all that money.

If all of us become vegan, we would invert the pyramid – we could all be healthy, we could all be wealthy and we could all be wise, and the health care issue would become the nonissue it really is anyway.

Man As Cancer

Man does not own this planet, but rather the planet owns man. This is a truth. To truly grasp the problems of health care, as well as to be able to formulate solutions, an adjustment of our current perspective is in order. Are the various diseases known as cancer the real problem, or is man the "cancer" and, therefore, the real problem?

Disease is not an automatic pitfall of the human condition. Diseases are caused by external influences, such as viruses, bacteria and, as is recently being acknowledged, parasites. Not all of these external influences are bad. Some, in fact, are essential to our continued well-being. For example, vitamin B12 is beneficial to both man and animals and is produced by a "good" bacteria. Streptococcus, on the other hand, can cause very painful sore throats, fever, etc. It is "bad" bacteria. Let us clearly understand that it is only man's perspective of bacteria that currently determines whether we call it good or bad. Though you may have never considered it before, it is fair to say the streptococcus bacteria don't think themselves "bad." In the case of a strep throat, we may take penicillin, another "good" bacteria, to rid ourselves of the bad bacteria.

Here, then, is another way of looking at cancer, or at least what we have come to look upon as cancer. A flesh-eating lifestyle is a cancer in the making, literally and metaphorically.

Thus far, this book has shown that love, truth, instinct and our very own physiology tell us to be vegan. Living opposite to love, truth, instinct and physiology is problematic. Cancer is a problem. Moreover, a world engaged in producing flesh actually creates more bad bacteria, which thrive on dead flesh. Conversely, a vegan diet minimizes bad bacteria, maximizes good bacteria and continually supports life.

There are some who believe man was given dominion over this planet. Dominion is still not the final authority, the dominion-giver is. When those with dominion (man) *choose* to live in contrast to principles (such as truth and love) clearly set down to guide us in our dominionship, we, in effect, become the cancer. What we currently perceive to be cancer may very well be the planet's cure for a deadly parasite – us.

Imagine if the police were asked to guard a bank and they chose instead to use their weapons to rob that bank. In this example we can clearly see that this is not only a problem but it is problematic – it is a problem that creates lots of other problems. To start with, whom does the bank call for help?

When it comes to man and cancer, our intellectuals and politicians can discuss health care until they're blue in the face, and they will go around and around and around. But until such time that there is a realignment with basic principles of humanity, intellect based upon humanity and some adept problem solving, man remains the biggest threat to the planet's survival and to the final authority's clear scheme of things. Man has a distinctive ability to allow cancer to be cancer or to choose to be the cancer. It is an amazing power we have, and we can use it or abuse it. At this point in time, in man's flesh-eating society, we've become the bank robbers with a badge, the cancer the planet needs to purge in order to function as it's supposed to. Flesh-eating man is clearly the bad bacteria threatening the planet's very survival. What flesh eaters currently perceive to be cancer may very well be the planet's antidote to its cataclysmic implosion.

Step back.

If the disease known as cancer can be seen as a parasite that feeds off man, it is actually dooming itself, because when its host eventually dies, so too will the parasite. So why doesn't cancer smarten up and help its host rather than harm it? The answer might simply be – cancer does what cancer does. It simply follows its biological imperative. A powerful distinction can now be made for man, who has no such biological imperative to destroy the planet, yet is doing so at an alarming pace. Folks, if we doom the planet, we doom ourselves. Are we not smarter than cancer? Man has a choice to be the parasite bringing about an eventual implosion or to be the planet's caretaker – and, as a natural consequence, our own caretaker.

The great news is that choosing a vegan way of life is also choosing to be the proper stewards of the land, its inhabitants, ourselves and our health care. And in VeganWorld, health care becomes the nonissue it really is anyway.

Now ask yourself what all the fuss is about health care. It is nothing short of a parasite's folly.

Chapter 16

Nutritional Mythology

W e now know that meat and dairy cannot exist in paradise and, therefore, are not in any way necessary for health. The meat and dairy industries, however, need you to believe the fallacy that you have to eat their products to obtain proper nutrition, e.g. adequate protein and calcium. If beef is high in protein and milk is high in calcium, from where does the cow get its protein or its calcium? The answer to this question offers tremendous insight into nutrition and the myths surrounding it.

Milk Does A Body Good (If You Happen To Be A Baby Cow)

Milk is truly a wonder food and, in some ways, it is nature at its finest. It contains protein, calcium and several vitamins, including the elusive B12. Cow's milk does do great things for a body – if that body happens to be a baby cow. One of its more notable qualities is that milk can quadruple the weight of a calf in a very short amount of time. If you want to put on a lot of weight and look like a cow, drink milk. But even then, you would need to concern yourself with several issues aside from obesity.

Firstly, the milk that is widely available in stores today is no longer just milk. Most of it contains heavy doses of hormones that are pumped into cows to make them produce more and more milk. Plus, thanks to the Byzantine biotechnology industry, some milk sold in stores is being produced by way of genetically engineered hormones. Without a clue as to the long-term effects on the lives of animals, humans and the planet, genetically engineered substances are increasingly making their way into the mass market. Cancer is on the rise and birth defects are rampant, the companies manufacturing these ingredients are wealthy and they keep saying it is perfectly safe to consume these foods. Anyone who doesn't think there's a connection might also be interested in buying one of my other lovely bridges that are for sale – cheap.

Secondly, a cow is designed to produce milk for a baby calf, not to supply milk to millions of thirsty people. This forced production of huge quantities by way of hormone injections causes severe stress to the cows and often produces infections such as mastitis which, in turn, causes the milk to potentially contain large amounts of pus. Pus consists of bacteria and white corpuscles that the cow produces in response to the infection.

Thirdly, not to allow profits to be outdone by disease, dairy farmers inject their cows with huge quantities of antibiotics to fight off diseases. Without antibiotics, many of these cows would die from the strain of producing so much milk. What's worse, over time the infections grow immune to the antibiotics and the cows need ever-increasing dosages to do the same work. But bacteria are smarter than they appear, and can mutate in response to antibiotics until they become resistant. Drinking milk containing all these antibiotics does the same thing to the bacteria in the human body. Increasingly, people are contracting antibiotic resistant infections, and a great deal of this can be due to the animal products being consumed. Drinking milk may very well be the worst thing you can do to your body.

For a fleeting moment, however, let's say that milk is as pure as the driven snow, such as is claimed by producers of organic milk. The question still remains, why should we drink milk at all? All mammals can digest the sugar in milk (lactose) as babies. Most, including humans, lose that ability as adults, as milk is no longer a dietary requirement. Rather than lactose intolerance being a problem in humans, it is the natural state of being.

Not only should adults avoid cow's milk, but so should babies. Human mother's milk is less likely than formula to cause diarrhea, constipation, respiratory infections, ear infections, urinary tract infections and allergies. Furthermore, studies have shown that feeding a baby mother's milk instead of formula lowers their risk of leukemia.

It is a strange fact that humans are just about the only species on the planet that drinks milk from another species. Dairy producers make consumers believe that milk is food. The real hard, bottom-line truth, however, is that milk is drunk because there is money to be made; just another integer in the equation of The Big Lie. In truth, humans should avoid milk at all costs.

Little White Lies

One of the dairy industry's perennial exhortations is that people should drink milk to obtain necessary protein. However, most people living in developed countries actually consume far too much protein already. Early in his career, T. Colin Campbell, author of *The China Study,* discovered that he could turn off cancer growth in animals simply by reducing their protein intake levels. But what is even more startling is that, upon further study, he found that not all proteins had the same effect. Casein, which makes up eighty-seven percent of cow's milk protein, consistently and strongly promoted all stages of cancer development, whereas proteins obtained from plants, including wheat and soy, did not promote cancer at all, even at higher levels of intake.

The human requirements for protein can easily be obtained from plants, the way nature intended. Big, strong, muscular bulls packed with protein don't consume meat or milk.

Some people claim to drink milk to obtain calcium for their bones. Consider that 100 grams of milk contain 116 milligrams of calcium, whereas 100 grams of garbanzo beans contain 150 milligrams of calcium, 100 grams of dried figs contain 126 milligrams of calcium, and 100 grams of broccoli contain 103 milligrams of calcium. Some vegetables contain more calcium than others, but virtually all vegetables have calcium, and often more than milk. In addition, the calcium in milk is not easily absorbed because other elements necessary for proper absorption are not present or in balance. Conversely, calcium obtained from plant foods is very easily and readily absorbed as plants contain the necessary chemical balance as well as many enzymes that are absolutely essential to a healthy body.

Down The Drain

As shown, drinking milk (and eating other animal products) will supply your body with far too much unabsorbable protein. Much of this protein is excreted in urine, creating still more problems. The kidneys require calcium to cleanse this excess protein out of your body. This calcium is often drawn out of your bones. Over time, this assists in the onset of osteoporosis: thin, weak and brittle bones. Drinking milk can actually facilitate osteoporosis, not prevent it, as the dairy producers would have us believe. Give it a few years and this will likely become a "new" finding. The Recommended Daily Allowance (RDA), unfortunately, is not generated by selfless Samaritans, so let the buyer beware.

Remember, huge and muscular mammals, such as cows, elephants, giraffes and horses, naturally maintain their bodies solely on grasses and other plants. The human body, also herbivorous by nature, can easily obtain all the protein it needs from plant foods.

A Tall, Cold Glass Of ...

Now think about milk in a way you may never have before. Think about what cow's milk really is – a glandular secretion nature intended for cows to produce so calves can put on weight fast. Think about where it comes from, the inside of a cow. If a cow sneezed on your food, would you eat it? Probably not. So why drink a different secretion of a cow (which, by the way, also contains mucus)? Milk from a mother to her baby is a wonder of nature. Milk from a cow to a human is an aberration. Aberrations beget aberrations.

So now think about why you really drink milk (or consume any dairy products). Is it because you think it's good for you? If so, why is that? Television commercials, perhaps? Well, gee. Why are there television commercials promoting milk? Is it that there are a bunch of selfless people out there engaging in the never-ending pursuit of your good health? Are these altruistic saints willing to spend millions upon millions of advertising dollars just for you to be healthy? Or is it that there are billions of dollars to be made by you drinking milk despite the consequences?

Health Or Corruption

You started drinking milk because that's what Mom gave you. She said it would help you grow up to be big and strong. But unless your mother is a true expert on nutrition, she is unlikely to fully understand the consequences. She is only following what her mother told her and what her mother told her before that, and they were all influenced by the marketing dollars spent by the milk peddlers.

Putting the nutritional drawbacks of drinking milk aside, almost all dairy cows live a very different life from the cheery images we are shown. Most live an extremely brutal existence, enclosed in small pens, chemically forced to produce more and more milk and, when their spent bodies can do no more, even with the assistance of Monsanto and other chemical companies, they are sent to slaughter. Because of the toll the continual forced milk production takes on their bodies many of these cows often can't stand up for their last ride to the slaughterhouse, so they're dragged, literally. These are called "downers" by the kind and caring folks in the industry, and because they are just products to them, they can lay there for hours in agony before being slaughtered. Many of the popular fast-food chains get their meat from these sources. The meal produced is anything but "Happy." The idea that drinking milk is not hurting cows is a fallacious one.

The truth is we drink milk out of habit and indoctrination, not because we need it to be healthy. Try using one of the many brands of soy milk readily available in supermarkets now. Use these for two weeks instead of cow's milk and you'll never go back. Leave the cow's milk for the baby cows. You'll be healthier and happier, and so will the cows.

The Incredible, Not-So-Edible Egg

Eggs serve a very distinct role in nature – to perpetuate the life of a species. For humans to eat eggs is a man-made aberration of nature. There is no reason or need to eat eggs, other than to perpetuate The Big Lie. Conversely, there are many reasons to avoid eggs.

Humanitarian issues aside for the moment, eating eggs provides the human body with many things the body would be better off not having. As with milk, eggs are naturally produced to further the species, not to provide breakfast to billions of people. As a result, the egg-laying chickens trying to keep up with our insatiable appetites are pumped with hormones and antibiotics, and are kept in conditions that force them to lay more eggs than nature intended, creating great stress in their bodies. Eating eggs means eating stress hormones, artificial growth hormones, fat and cholesterol. So why eat them, other than for reasons attributed to The Big Lie? The truth is, eating eggs has many drawbacks and no benefits.

An Egg Is ... An Egg

Think about what an egg really is. It is an unfertilized (for the most part), gelatinous chicken fetus waiting to happen. An egg (the food) is actually an egg (an ovum with the potential for becoming a chicken fetus). How anybody could sit down to eat an egg and then get upset if a fly lands on the plate is an amazing phenomenon that offers insight into the animal product eater's corrupt conditioning.

And, of course, egg-laying chickens, like milk-producing cows, live a life very different from the cheery images we are shown by the meat and dairy industries. Most are kept in cages so small that they literally cannot even turn around, and in order to keep them from killing themselves and each other their beaks are sliced off as a matter of routine.

Protein

Protein is nothing more than a collection of amino acids. Eggs contain protein, but so do carrots and broccoli and pasta and rice and beans and nuts. Proteins are present in all animal and vegetable matter. By eating a wide variety of plant foods you can ensure adequate protein intake. It's really as simple as that. Cows, horses, elephants, and giraffes get plenty of protein, and they don't sneak a protein shake or a hamburger when no one is looking.

Choices

Eating meat and dairy products provides fat, cholesterol and a host of other malady makers. As a result, in addition to protein and calcium, eating meat and dairy can provide us with:

1. Heart disease	8. Obesity
2. High blood pressure	9. Environmental catastrophe
3. Colon cancer	10. Monumental cruelty and brutality
4. Diabetes (adult onset)	11 Control-hungry regimes
5. Gout and arthritis	12 Sociopathy
6. Osteoporosis	13. Distance from God
7. Kidney disease	14. Greeting cards referring to paradise

In contrast, eating plant foods gives us protein, calcium, vitamins, minerals, phytochemicals and enzymes essential for bodily health. In fact, the more plant foods you eat the more nutrients your body gets. In addition to complete nutrition, eating a plant-based diet can provide us with:

1. Homeostasis	8 Freedom
2. Natural weight control	9. Love
3. Bodily health	10. Drinkable water/breathable air
4. Soundness of mind and spirit	11. Respect
5. Truth	12. Humanity
6. Compassion	13. Paradise and a connection to God
7. Peace	14. Oneness and kinship with the world and all that is just, decent and holy

So, which is objectively intelligent, wise, humane and truly healthy, an animal-based diet or a plant-based diet?

The New Millennium

Hardly a day goes by that we don't hear about how soybeans can prevent cancer or how oatmeal can lower cholesterol, etc. When was the last time you heard that beef or chicken prevent hypertension or heart disease? Plant and vegetable foods can prevent and even reverse these and other widespread maladies. While science is slowly realizing these elementary basic truths, they have yet to make the direct connection. Yes, the scientific community now says soybeans can prevent cancer, and in different studies they say eating meat causes cancer, but they haven't yet publicly made the direct (and obvious) connection. It is still very political, after all, and meat and dairy is still the financial backbone of government and its research.

Can you imagine what would occur if you not only ate soybeans but avoided meat and dairy? What do you think would happen to your chances of getting cancer? Can you imagine if the whole world ate this way? Cancer can be utterly defeated, and not by the brute force of money and drugs, but by the wisdom of humanity. It is the latter that exclusively holds the "cure."

Meat Is Flesh

What is termed in the common vernacular "meat," the neatly packaged stuff in your local supermarket, is really the flesh and blood of an animal. When you eat flesh, you are also eating blood, urine, hormones (naturally produced by the animal), stress and fear hormones (produced by the slaughtering of the animal or the suffocating of the fish), artificial or genetically engineered growth hormones and antibiotics (injected into many animals), mercury (in fish from polluted water), and the list goes on and on, depending upon the particular animal product.

Some people get really disgusted if they find a fly or a hair on their hamburger. After becoming vegan, they'll wonder why the hair is any more disgusting than the flesh out of which the hair grows. Why is the body of a fly any more disgusting than the body parts of murdered cows? You don't have to step back too far for this answer – it lies in corrupt conditioning and denial. At least in the case of the fly, it will usually land on your plate of its own volition.

Never has a cow or a pig or a chicken walked up and sat on someone's dinner plate of its own free will.

The Elusive Truth About Vitamin B12

In contrast to meat, plant foods are pure and complete nutrition. They contain protein, carbohydrates, necessary fat, calcium, fiber, many phytochemicals essential for a healthy body, all the necessary minerals, as well as the entire spectrum of vitamins, with one notable exception. Vitamin B12, which is necessary for the synthesis of red blood cells and the maintenance of the nervous system, is not found in most plant foods. It is, however, found in meat, eggs and dairy. This is often cited as proof that humans need to consume animal products. A deeper understanding of vitamin B12 is in order.

B12 is produced by bacteria found in soil. When a cow grazes it ingests some soil clinging to the roots of the grass. It is from this ingested soil that the cow's flesh and milk get their B12. Likewise, man could get his B12 by eating unprocessed foods that are grown in the soil, like carrots and potatoes, assuming they were grown naturally. Relax. You do not have to eat soil. Even washed carrots will have minute traces of B12, and the amount of B12 the human body needs is smaller than any other known vitamin. Further, some data shows that B12 is found in fermented soy products, yeast, sprouts and sea vegetables.

In reality, most of today's produce is grown in soil that has been depleted of its nutrients. The culprit is a meat-producing world. For this reason it may not be a bad idea to eat foods fortified with vitamin B12 or take a supplement. In VeganWorld this would not be necessary.

Eat meat and you can get E.Coli. Eat carrots and you can get B12. Don't rob B12 from the animals, there's plenty of it for everyone at the source.

Against Life

It is also important to know that in healthy animals, including humans, bacterial B12 can (and should) be found in the gut and mouth. However, the "foods" we *shouldn't* be eating play a part in reducing the efficacy of this natural source of B12.

The antibiotics ingested from eating animals, as well as those we ingest as a result of our disease care system, mean that we no longer have the natural bacterial makeup that we should, or once had. The antibiotics are not "smart bombs," so they kill good bacteria, such as those that produce B12, along with any bad bacteria. Eating meat, therefore, creates an unnatural chemistry in our bodies that prevents us from hosting enough of our own natural B12. To suggest that we need to eat meat in order to obtain enough B12 is like saying that we need to eat meat in order to prevent heart disease.

Even cows are having trouble obtaining enough natural B12, as animal agriculture has decimated our soil's composition. Routine B12 injections solve this problem very well. The laboratory that does nutritional analysis of meat and dairy can't tell where the B12 is coming from. We just hear meat and dairy contain vitamin B12.

We live in a meat-eating world, so disease will not vanish overnight. But as you become vegan, you may very well get sick less often, requiring fewer antibiotics, which, in turn, will help you to get sick less often still.

When I went for my blood test to get my marriage license I mentioned to the doctor that I didn't eat meat. Thinking he was being helpful, he began listing things I should be careful of, such as insufficient B12 and calcium. I wonder if he tells people who eat meat that they should be careful of heart disease and cancer. Somehow I doubt it. How many people died from a vitamin B12 deficiency this year? In round numbers, zero. How many people died from heart disease and cancer this year? In round numbers, 1,500,000 in the United States alone.

Get With The Program

Veganism is quite possibly the best lifestyle improvement you could ever make. You may not only be immensely healthier, but you will also be contributing to a safe and sane planet. Please notice, I said safe and sane, not safer and saner. There's a huge difference. The latter is the attempt, while the former, the one vegans effect, is the achievement.

A Weak Stereotype

It is possible to become vegan and lose too much weight, in part because a vegan diet typically contains fewer calories and fat than a meat-based diet. These few people (and opportunistic meat industry advertising agencies) are probably responsible for the stereotype of thin and weak vegetarians. If someone were to give up all food with the exception of licorice sticks and water he would be vegan, but he would not be very healthy. The other side of the equation is also true. The person who eats nothing but hamburgers and fried chicken is … well, I don't know what he's called, but he's equally, if not more, unhealthy, and usually a lot fatter.

Most vegans are not only healthier than their meat-eating counterparts, but usually have far more stamina and strength. There are Olympic and professional athletes who are vegan (or vegetarian), but most people aren't aware of this because McDonald's and Kentucky Fried Chicken don't sponsor sporting events that promote the virtues of not eating dead animals.

> *"My best year of track competition was the first year I ate a vegan diet."* – Carl Lewis, Olympic Gold medalist

You may wonder why the soybean or carrot industries, for example, don't promote this message. Several years ago I produced and hosted a radio show called *Vegetarian Lifestyles*, and I contacted these industries thinking they would be great sponsors. I was about to further my education. As it turns out, the vast majority of vegetable crops are sold to the animal industries for livestock feed. Moreover, as if that wasn't enough of an education, I learned that some produce businesses are owned by companies also vested in animal product industries. They refused to participate.

Remember to *remove* animal foods and *replace* them with plant foods. To simply eliminate animal foods without eating adequate plant foods in their stead is to deprive your body of the caloric fuel and nutrition it needs to run. The point, then, is to maintain a vegan diet that is varied, tasty, satisfying and nutritious. In doing so, you are increasing your chances for a healthy life many, many times over. Not only will you probably be much healthier, but your quality of life will soar. Yes, your caloric intake will be reduced simply by substituting vegetable products for animal products, but you shouldn't be concerned about getting insufficient calories. It has been proven in numerous studies that "caloric restricted" diets utilized over a lifetime drastically increase lifespan.

The Balancing Act

In an attempt to justify eating meat, some people will insist that everything is okay in balance or in moderation. Such a statement sounds so reasonable that it seems it could not possibly be just another part of The Big Lie. In reality, this balancing act is the essence of subjectivity.

Someone who eats three hamburgers a day may consider moderation to mean one hamburger a day. On the other hand, to someone who never eats any animal products, eating even one ounce of salmon could not possibly be considered moderation. Subjective moderation is relative to one's customary methods, but offers virtually nothing in the way of true, healthy, natural eating (and living). In fact, it is very dangerous, as it facilitates a belief that one is living in balance, which is still more fuel for The Big Lie. Then, people who have "cut down" don't understand why they are still contracting illnesses and diseases, as they believe they are living in balance. But whether they believe it or not, eating animal products in any amount is not a balanced diet at all, it is only a balancing act.

To Debate Or Not To Debate

The debate on issues of health, disease, nutrition and malnutrition will rage on for years because they are not being approached from a standpoint of truth, but rather subjectivity. Health and disease, nutrition and malnutrition are nothing more than the effect of living with or in contrast to nature. Until this truth is embraced, nonsensical diet fads will come and go, and confusion will reign supreme.

These days, science recognizes fat as a leading cause of various diseases. This can lead one to surmise that by eating meats and other animal products low in fat that you're safe from these diseases. This can be very dangerous conjecture. When a "product" that nature never intended us to ingest is ingested, it is utterly problematic. Just because fat is now recognized by the scientific community as unhealthy does not mean there are not other elements in unnatural foods that are equally, if not more, unhealthy. Science has just not gotten to these yet. In fact, it may very well be animal protein that is the most carcinogenic substance of all.

Remember, if someone tricks you into eating paint it doesn't then mean that paint is food. Animals and their parts, with or without fat, are not food for human beings and cannot ever be made safe or healthy for human ingestion. Plants and their parts are exclusively what nature, and even God, has provided to humans for food.

The Food Chain

The food chain is commonly thought of as a sequence of plants and animals in a community, in which each member feeds on the member below it, with man on top of the whole eerie pyramid. This "circle of life" is often referred to in an attempt to justify man's meat-eating ways. However, this concept is nothing more than yet another cog in The Big Lie. In fact, the modern-day concept of the food chain is not a truth used to explain natural life, but rather a fabrication, or subjective truth, born from an unnatural life, used to justify that unnatural life.

Post hoc ergo propter hoc. It is an easy assumption to think that merely because one thing happens after another that the latter is a result of the former. This is a very dangerous assumption. Man engaging in the practice of eating animals and then citing this practice as evidence that man is on top of the food chain is nothing more than subjective justification. Over time, this can seem to be a truth, but, again, it is just another vital cog in The Big Lie.

> *"Truly man is the king of beasts, for his brutality exceeds theirs."* – Leonardo da Vinci

Let's say a man secretly puts a bomb in a car and then detonates it. He then says to his friend, while pointing at the blown-up car, "See? I told you cars explode." Is the statement in and of itself true? Yes, it is. But it is very misleading. The whole truth is that cars don't explode unless we blow them up. The bomb maker's friend, not knowing the whole truth, may very well believe that cars just simply explode and will then spread what he believes to be true to others. Over time, the mistaken belief can become an accepted societal "truth."

The food chain concept is no different. It is a fallacious belief born out of an unnatural and inhumane lifestyle in an attempt to justify that lifestyle. It is a circular argument: We eat meat, *therefore* we are at the top of the food chain. Then: We eat meat *because* we are at the top of the food chain. Absurd! Even more absurd when you consider that man's physiology is designed to eat at the lowest level of the food chain, i.e. plants. More absurd still when you consider that if this supposed food chain were accurate and man were on top, as the meat eater's paradigm suggests, man would eat lions and coyotes (cats and dogs), not cows and chickens.

Nature intended humans to be vegan, yet most humans spend their existence rejecting this truth. Rejecting nature's truths is the very reason the world, its people, animals and ecosystems are being destroyed from the inside out. This supposed food chain, and man's position therein, is not a truth at all. It is an essential element to keeping The Big Lie alive, and the Earth and all its parts in grave peril.

Truth, love, instinct, basic human physiology and humanity are some of the strongest chains in nature's order, and are the food chain's weakest links.

Choice Or Compulsion

A compulsion, according to *Webster's New World Dictionary*, is "an irresistible, repeated, irrational impulse to perform some act." The same dictionary offers many definitions of the word "choice," including "implies the chance, right, or power to choose, usually by free exercise of one's judgment." Clearly, choice and compulsion are diametrically opposed.

There is nothing healthy, intelligent or humane about eating animals and animal products, but The Big Lie creates a lifelong compulsion to consume these items. Whilst society lives in accordance with The Big Lie, disease, inhumanity, blindness and monumental stupidity will reign supreme under the guise of civilization. Conversely, *choosing* a diet based on health, intelligence and humanity cannot possibly include meat and animal products.

Choice is a tremendous gift and responsibility. Make a choice between cruelty and humanity, darkness and enlightenment, disease and health, lies and truth. Meat eaters live by compulsion; vegans live by choice. Once you begin consciously choosing between choice and compulsion, winning the battle may now be just a matter of time.

"Better than a man who conquers a thousand times a thousand men, is he who conquers himself. He is the mightiest of warriors."   – The Buddha

Chapter 17

Health & Disease

"I became vegetarian because it was the right thing to do, not because I thought it would protect me from certain diseases or extend my lifespan ... If new studies reveal tomorrow that the four food groups were dead-on accurate after all and that 2-3 servings of meat per day really are necessary to maintain maximum health, I'll be disappointed. But I'll still be vegan."

– Obligate Carnivore, by Jed Gillen

Many people first think of healthy eating when they hear the "V" word. Veganism is healthy, but by now you should see the larger picture. Sociopathic, self-serving concepts of health will steer you the wrong way. Yes, a vegan diet can help you to permanently lose weight and help prevent and reverse high blood pressure, diabetes, heart disease, etc., etc. Studies suggest it will even increase your life span. These are all benefits of being vegan. So what?

In order for mankind to move forward, it is vital to understand that health is a product of all the topics we've been discussing – love, humanity, truth, etc. – not the other way around. Part of the problem is that once a society is engaged in meat eating and production, those caught up in it will find any means to justify what they do.

"Enough research will tend to support your theory."
                        – Unknown

The plethora of bad information about healthy diets has gotten so dizzying because everyone has heard someone say, "Oh, boy. It doesn't matter what I eat or drink because everything causes cancer, even tap water." Research be damned. The truth is, everything doesn't cause cancer (or obesity or heart disease). Carrots do not cause cancer; apples do not cause cancer; beans do not cause cancer; wheat does not cause cancer. Even products made from plants, such as veggie burgers, don't cause cancer. In parts of the world where people eat no meat or dairy, there is little or no cancer. Sure, the pesticides we spray on crops cause all types of problems, but most pesticide ingestion does not come from eating plants. Eighty percent of all pesticides are applied to crops that are used as feed for cattle and other animals headed for human consumption. By eating the flesh of an animal, you're eating concentrated pesticides from everything the animal has eaten over the course of its life. By abstaining from meat consumption you automatically, and drastically, reduce your pesticide ingestion. Eat organically grown plant-based foods and we go back to the truth that carrots do not cause cancer. In fact, they can prevent it. Much to the chagrin of the animal product industries, what's becoming harder and harder to deny is that plant foods can even reverse disease, disease that is created almost solely from animal products.

Drinking tap water may, in fact, cause cancer. That's why even vegans can develop cancer. Remember, however, that it's not the water that's causing the problem, but rather what we have put into the water as a result of our unnatural eating and lifestyle habits. Chemical runoff from huge animal farming corporations seeping into our drinking water supply has led to many reports of carcinogens in our tap water. Moreover, there is now compelling evidence that it is actually the protein from animal products that prevents the human body from naturally fighting off cancer.

It is no longer a secret that eating meat causes cancer. The only thing most scientists seem to still be arguing about is just how many cancers are caused by meat and animal products. Further, a world engaged in meat production causes cancer (and obesity and hypertension and diabetes and heart disease and ...).

> *"The beef industry has contributed to more American deaths than all the wars of this century, all natural disasters, and all automobile accidents combined."*
> – Dr. Neal Barnard, President,
> Physicians Committee for Responsible Medicine

The Epidemic Of Obesity

People of all countries in which meat is the centerpiece of the diet are overweight. It is a global epidemic. Everywhere you look you see fat people. Even children are becoming dangerously overweight in ever-increasing numbers, and being overweight can be horrible for them for a lot of reasons. Being fat is unhealthy physically, mentally and emotionally. Overweight kids can't run or play as they should, their social lives are affected by their weight, and all of this has enormous impact on their self-esteem and self-image.

Have you ever met, or even heard of, a morbidly obese vegan? It is interesting how widespread (no pun intended) the obesity problem is and yet very few people ever make the proper connection. Let's get one thing perfectly clear: Nobody is fat solely because of a "glandular problem" or any of the other reasons you may hear. It may be true that some people are blessed with an ability to eat as much as they want without gaining an ounce, while others merely have to glance at a doughnut to put on five pounds at the hips.

That's just the way life is. Tiger Woods is a great golfer; I can't win a game of miniature golf. You've got to work with what you've got.

While there are "genetic propensities," more often than not our propensity is nothing more than us tending to live and eat like our parents. If our parents were sedentary and ate all the wrong foods, we, too, often become sedentary and follow their poor dietary lead. As a result, we are usually affected by the same diseases and conditions as our parents, leading some people to make a genetic connection. To go beyond that is, in all too many cases, a flagrant cop-out.

How many people in the Nazi concentration camps were fat? Of the millions who were in those gruesome places, surely one of them must have had a "slow metabolism" or "glandular problems," yet not a fat one among them – categoric proof that lifestyle and environment override genetic propensity.

In an attempt to show that eating animal products is not responsible for obesity, some will point to the one person in a million who eats nothing but hamburgers and ice cream and never gains an ounce. Some people win the lottery. But most lose. For every one that wins, how many millions die trying? There are just enough winners to keep the fallacy alive.

Some people are born fat and get fatter, others are the proper weight as babies and children, and then get fatter as they get older. The reason is simple: meat and animal products hinder metabolism. Further, most people easily ingest over 600 calories by eating half a pound of beef in a hamburger. To take in the same number of calories from, say, carrots, you would have to eat about 3.5 pounds of them. Just try eating that many carrots! Even if you could, you'd be getting a tremendous amount of healthy vitamins, minerals, enzymes and phytochemicals, whereas with meat you're eating fat, blood, hormones and antibiotics. Even "conventional" nutritionists and doctors recommend eating as many fruits and vegetables as you want. The recommendation is always prefaced by saying eat "at least" several servings. Conversely, for meat, the recommendation is "not more than" a few ounces.

Sure, some people become sedentary over the years, contributing to their weight gain, but that's also a result of poor food choices. Vegans generally do not gain weight as they age, certainly not nearly as much as their meat-eating counterparts, and the activity levels of vegans do not decline as drastically as they age.

No matter how well-intentioned they may be, most diets are a waste of time, and are even counterproductive, to the extent that temporary deprivation is not the solution to being overweight and can actually contribute to it. Dieting adversely affects the metabolism, which invariably results in weight gain. Anyone who has ever had a weight problem knows the perpetual roller coaster ride of fatdom. Dieting is the folly of a meat-eating world. If you are overweight and become vegan, the chances of you staying overweight are slim (no pun intended). Veganism is a diet that does not require counting calories, fat grams or reading volumes of diet books. Veganism is the ultimate diet.

Recently, some diet schemes have been advocating eating *only* meat. This is such a dangerous proposition and can wreak enormous damage to the human body. The buildup of ketones and cholesterol, to name two, is why even the proponents don't advocate this diet for extended periods. (Ketones are chemicals produced by the liver when the body cannot use glucose and must break down fat for energy. They can poison and even kill body cells.) Perhaps not coincidentally, Dr. Robert Atkins, the main proponent of one of these high protein diets, suffered a heart attack, congestive heart failure and hypertension before the fall that caused his death, although we may never know whether these conditions precipitated the fall, as the family did not permit an autopsy.

Because of the way the human body responds to such a regimen, some people may temporarily lose weight. Ultimately, however, because all diets destroy natural metabolism, for every pound dieters lose, they may very well gain two or three back. Additionally, over time, their bodies will pay an even higher price, like the car whose gas tank is full of paint.

Vegans are generally slim throughout their lives, and they also generally don't diet. It is odd that vegans are often stereotyped as being thin, and yet obese people say they've tried "every" diet. Apparently, they've only tried every diet that includes animal parts.

Fat Is As Fat Does

The overweight epidemic is painfully widespread amongst children, and while I was attending the National Food Policy Conference there was a workshop and lecture on this problem. More and more children are overweight and no one seems to know why. I sat and listened to a panel of thoroughly schooled and experienced experts try to address this epidemic. One psychologist (with a list of credentials so long even I was impressed with how someone so educated could be so stupid) discussed eating disorders and how they apply to obesity in children. This expert went so far as to offer a verbose and complicated comparison between alcoholism and obesity. She explained that in the case of alcoholism the offending product can be removed entirely. But with obesity, you must *modify* your food because you can't remove it completely. Her choice of words intrigued me, specifically her choice of the word "food."

During the question and answer session that followed her presentation I said, "In response to eating disorders, specifically dealing with obesity, Bunny (that's her name, honest) stated that, unlike alcohol, you cannot remove food entirely but must modify it. But meat and dairy are like paint, in that they are not fit for human consumption and can, and should be, removed from the diet entirely. Nobody is getting overweight from carrots, apples or even veggie burgers." Bunny readjusted herself in her seat, but offered nothing but five seconds of silence. I had their attention, so I continued. "My question is, have there been any official studies on vegetarian or vegan regimens and how they affect weight?"

There was nothing but silence for at least fifteen seconds. If it wasn't so sad, it would have been comical to watch this panel of "experts" look blankly back and forth at each other. Finally, one of the panelists (no, not Bunny) said quietly, "No, there haven't been any studies that we know of, though Dean Ornish has published a book dealing with that subject." (Dr. Ornish is a renowned cardiologist. His book, *Eat More, Weigh Less*, recommends a plant-based diet.)

I replied, "Exactly. And he has proven that you can actually eat more food and still lose weight."

The panel of experts seemed more bothered by the facts that they'd overlooked than they were happy to have been enlightened. A great realization struck me. No one, not even the so-called experts, is looking in the right place for solutions. How could they? They all eat meat, and most are backed by the meat and dairy industries. It is nothing short of bizarre that an overweight society pejoratively stereotypes vegans as thin but then spends untold dollars and resources looking for a solution to obesity.

Up to this very point, you may have never thought of meat as anything other than food. But meat is not food. The fact is, meat is death, and death begets death. This is not meant to be a dramatic statement, but in truth, eating meat turns a human stomach into a cemetery; and, for many people, a very large cemetery.

"We live by the death of others. We are burial places."
        – Leonardo da Vinci

Putting a child on a diet and beginning the lifelong roller coaster ride of obesity should be considered a crime. Putting a child on a diet while feeding him or her animal products is a crime worthy of the insanity defense. The only safe, reasonable, intelligent and humane solution is to remove all animal products from the menu. In doing so, weight control will become a nonissue.

Permanent Weight Control

The solution to the problem of obesity is very simple. For permanent weight control, don't eat less, eat more real food. Fruits, vegetables, grains, legumes, nuts and seeds are food, as are the many products made from them such as veggie burgers (but be careful, not all "veggie burgers" are *all* veggie – read the ingredients). As you begin eating this way, your metabolism can normalize, your energy level will most probably soar and your weight will take care of itself. Unless you eat bags of potato chips, loaves of bread or platefuls of French fries, you will most probably never, ever be on a diet again. You can completely forget about counting calories and you will not be obese.

Heart Disease

The problems caused by eating animals don't stop at the waistline. In fact, eating animal products is a primary factor, if not *the* factor, in many diseases.

Coronary artery blockages is the condition commonly known as heart disease. In simple terms, this is the buildup of fatty plaque inside the coronary arteries, and it kills over seven million people worldwide every year. That's one person every four seconds! It has gotten to the point where heart attacks are considered to be a normal part of the aging process. In truth, heart disease is not a normal part of the aging process at all, but rather an aberration caused by eating animal products, and the disease can begin with the very first swallow. It's a process that develops slowly over the years as we ingest animals. Autopsies on young soldiers killed in battle have shown that virtually one hundred percent of them have *at least* the visible beginnings of this disease, even those younger than twenty.

The buildup of fatty plaque inside the arteries comes primarily from cholesterol and saturated fat. Plant foods contain zero cholesterol and usually very little saturated fat, while animal products are loaded with both. (Saturated fat can be identified as fat that remains solid at room temperature.)

Don't allow yourself to be misled by companies trying to sell cholesterol-lowering drugs that say high cholesterol is a natural event. Of course they want you to believe that; they want you to be powerless, which will help them sell more product. Let the buyer beware. Cholesterol is a natural substance manufactured by the liver and is an essential element to our bodies. Cholesterol is not the enemy. The problem begins, however, when your body is inundated by additional cholesterol and saturated fats from the animal parts you are eating. Then, slick advertising campaigns orchestrated by pharmaceutical companies want you to believe that you simply have bad genetics and the solution is their handy-dandy statin drug. Interestingly, while they want you to believe their pills are the cure-all to your problem, there is usually a small print disclaimer that these drugs have not been shown to prevent heart attacks. Again, let the buyer beware.

> *"A third of the food we eat keeps us alive. The other two-thirds keeps the doctors alive."* – Orson Welles

Even young children who eat the Standard American Diet (SAD), comprised of meat and dairy, can have the beginnings of heart disease. As the years go by and more animal products are ingested, more and more fatty plaque builds up, narrowing the openings of the arteries. After many SAD years the arteries can become completely clogged, leading to a heart attack or, if the arteries to the brain become clogged, a stroke.

> *"When you see the Golden Arches, you are probably on the road to the Pearly Gates."*   – Dr. William Castell,
> Director of Laboratories
> for the Framingham Heart Study

Forty Years In An Instant

A forty-year-old man who has just suffered a heart attack is rushed to the hospital, where he dies, and the doctors say he died of a "sudden" heart attack. Folks, there is nothing sudden about it. This heart attack took forty years to create. There are other factors that can contribute to a heart attack, such as stress, since stress can constrict the arteries. But these are usually just exacerbating factors. Imagine having your arteries clogged ninety percent with fatty plaque and then your blood vessels constrict another ten pecent because of stress. Clearly, you could withstand the stress if it wasn't for your animal fat-clogged arteries.

Radical Medicine

There are some doctors, such as Dr. Michael Klaper, Dr. Dean Ornish, Dr. Julian Whitaker and Dr. Neal Barnard, who are outspoken on the subject of proper prevention and reversal of heart disease. In fact, Dr. Ornish has proven heart disease can be reversed by way of a plant-based diet. Why do you suppose the medical community at large, and the American Medical Association (AMA) in particular, does not utilize their considerable resources to heavily promote this simple lifesaving technique? The truth is, there's more money in pushing drugs and surgery than there is in teaching people how to eat properly. Remember, buy one tomato and you can eat tomatoes for the rest of your life. It would be impossible to get a patent on tomatoes.

When Dr. Dean Ornish was about to release his irrefutable proof that heart disease can be prevented *and* reversed via a low-fat, plant-based diet, along with exercise and some relaxation techniques, the medical community was quick to blast him (the die-hard dimwits still do). They described his program as "radical." But think for a moment. Clear your mind of the misinformation that emanates from the medical community with which you have been indoctrinated and then ask yourself which of the following two examples is really radical?

1. Showing people how to eat healthily, how and why to exercise, and teaching them how to properly deal with stress.
2. Cutting open a living human being, sawing his bones apart, lifting most of his chest out of his body and re-routing the circulatory system, otherwise known as a heart bypass operation.

The radical truth is heart disease, for all intents and purposes, would be nonexistent in a vegan world. In fact, it already is in areas of the world that don't eat meat. Another radical truth, incidentally, is that in a vegan world cardiologists would have a radical reduction in income.

> *"Men dig their graves with their own teeth and die more by those fated instruments than the weapons of their enemies."*
> — Thomas Moffett

Hypertension

Another epidemic closely related to heart disease is hypertension, or high blood pressure, although few people realize what high blood pressure really is. As arteries become clogged and blood cannot circulate freely, pressure builds up behind the blockage. Think of when you put your thumb over the end of a garden hose. High blood pressure is essentially the same thing.

Everyone knows that high blood pressure and heart disease go hand in hand. Even the medical community states that people with high blood pressure are far more likely to die of a heart attack or stroke. Well, no kidding. What they're not telling you is high blood pressure is literally a heart attack in the making. High blood pressure is, in very simple terms, a byproduct of the progression of heart disease, when the arteries are clogged enough to slow the flow of blood, but not clogged enough to shut down the flow completely. Stress can also cause a rise in blood pressure, since stress can constrict the arteries. However, stress induced hypertension in and of itself is rarely much of a problem. It just exacerbates the real problem.

Become vegan and you may not develop any of the major degenerative and terminal illnesses. In fact, you can even reverse these illnesses. Yes, you will die, but it might be from something really unusual, such as old age. And, by the way, old age doesn't mean seventy or eighty years old. This is old age to a human body that has, over the course of its life, consumed animals and animal products and lived in a meat-producing world. Old age for a human body that has lived in accordance with nature in a world that has lived in accordance with nature has been estimated by some to be around 120 years old.

> *"We are the first to come up with a life-expectancy figure showing a very important increase in life expectancy for those who follow a vegetarian diet for a long period of time."*   – Dr. Pramil Singh,
>   Loma Linda University, California

It is obviously impossible to study the enormous, wide-ranging health benefits of what would happen to mankind if we all lived a vegan lifestyle in a vegan world. Notwithstanding this difficulty, the Nobel prize-winning author Isaac Bashevis Singer perhaps summed it up best when he was asked if you should be a vegetarian for health reasons. He replied, "Yes. For the health of the chicken!"

Diabetes

Insulin is a hormone secreted by the pancreas to help digest sugars, and diabetes is a disease in which the pancreas does not produce enough insulin, or the body cannot utilize the insulin efficiently. As a result, many people think that diabetics shouldn't eat sugar. This is something of a half-truth, and rather misleading. The actual problem is what is suppressing the body's ability to manufacture and use insulin. If you haven't already guessed, the culprit is, surprise, surprise, animal products.

The most common form of diabetes is adult-onset, or Type 2, which is often one of the easiest conditions to reverse. Many Type 2 diabetics can reduce, if not completely eliminate, their need for insulin injections when they become vegan. Avoiding sugar does little to correct the problem, other than perpetuate the need for doctor visits to get more insulin. Simply removing sugar from the diet of a meat-eating diabetic is a lot like attempting to cure a tree that is dying from lack of water by removing the brown leaves. Remove meat and animal parts from the diet along with overly processed products and the body will most likely normalize itself. I have heard diabetics say they shouldn't have an apple because of the sugar. Then they eat a piece of chicken. I never know whether to laugh or cry.

"An apple a day keeps the doctor away." – Unknown

Kidney Disease & Osteoporosis – Two For The Price Of One

Bone is made up, in part, of calcium atoms. These calcium atoms need phosphate atoms to bond together, helping to form a hard bone. Each phosphate atom has an extra electron that facilitates this bonding of calcium and phosphate onto the collagen fiber of the bone. Animal products contain high amounts of sulphur amino acids. When you eat animal products, your liver breaks down the protein into amino acid fragments and chains of hydrogen atoms. This broken-down protein enters the blood from the liver. As the blood circulates to the bone, these long chains of negatively charged hydrogen atoms (free radicals) enter the bone and rip the phosphate atoms off the bone so that they, themselves, may become electrically balanced. Once the phosphate atom is taken by the negatively charged hydrogen atom, the calcium atom can no longer bond to the collagen fiber of the bone. The calcium atom simply floats away in the blood, leading to, over time, osteoporosis.

Osteoporosis takes years to develop, but another common malady can be taking place in the interim. The calcium atoms that could no longer bond to the bone enter the bloodstream and circulate to the kidneys, where they collect and build up as stones. Many kidney stones come from one's own bone.

Osteoporosis and kidney disease result from diets containing high amounts of animal protein. As a result, drinking milk to get calcium may not be the solution you thought it was.

The High Cost Of Free Radicals

Free radicals have many causes, and some are completely natural. But many causes are not so natural – poor environment, carbon dioxide, stress, fatty foods and animal products. Eating a diet high in animal products turns the body's cellular structure into a war zone. In the simplest of terms, free radicals are negatively charged atoms in need of an electron to balance them out. So each free radical circulates through the body and steals an electron from a healthy, balanced cell. These cells, having been robbed of their electron, then become free radicals themselves.

Free radicals are a natural part of the body's process, but too many, caused by unnatural lifestyles, can weaken every cell in your body, and the continual weakening is responsible for the body succumbing to many diseases, including cancer.

Antioxidants

To combat this proliferation of free radicals we have the body's superheroes, antioxidants, which, in essence, chelate, or bond, with free radicals and carry them off into the waste matter, saving your healthy cells from destruction. Antioxidants are, for example, vitamins A, C and K, as well as thousands of phytochemicals, many of which science has yet to identify. Antioxidants are *abundant* in fruits and vegetables.

By abstaining from ingesting animal products, you greatly reduce the number of free radicals in your system. Then, by eating an abundance of plant foods, you supply your body with amazing preventative defenses in the way of antioxidants. Eating only animal products is practically suicide. Better, but not good, is to eat a combination of animals and plants. However, this creates a perpetual cellular battleground in your body, in which the war is usually lost to cancer. Eating an exclusively plant-based diet is not only the best way to eat from an ethically proper and moral standpoint, it is the only healthy way to eat. Eating this way provides the body with the tools it needs to maintain homeostasis, i.e. a healthy, harmonious being. Be vegan and you may even die of old age. Unfortunately, though, even vegans have to breathe the air and drink the water con-taminated by a meat-producing world, so no one is truly safe. This is not only a good reason to become vegan, but to get your family and friends – and enemies – to become vegan.

Cleaning It All Up

Eating meat has an unlimited supply of drawbacks, while eating plant foods has an unlimited supply of benefits, another of which is fiber. Fiber, which is absent in animal products and abundant in plant foods, scrubs the walls of the large intestine and colon, keeping them clean.

When animal products are consumed, a fatty film builds up on the walls of the intestines and colon, inhibiting nutrients from getting through (most of the absorption of nutrients takes place in the intestines). Over time, as more animal products are ingested, this film thickens and coats the intestinal walls and becomes a breeding ground for various parasites and worms. This film not only prevents nutrients from being absorbed but facilitates the growth of polyps and tumors.

Eating plant foods along with animal foods is better than not eating plant foods at all, but is not enough to prevent or clean the colon of this deadly film. An exclusively plant-based diet is the only way to a clean colon. When someone gives up eating animal foods, the fiber from the plant foods helps to scrub away this rotting, fatty matter. In time, this person can return to what should be a normal state and will, again, be absorbing plenty of nutrients.

"You Are What You Eat" Is Only Half A Saying

The bottom line is that everything we put in our mouths becomes the essence of our cellular structure. But there is another important fact to be remembered – you are what you don't excrete! Everything that does not come out becomes a part of your body. Do you want the fat and blood of animals to be a permanent fixture inside you? If you don't want animal fat permanently lining your arterial and intestinal walls, the answer is simple: become vegan. If having this stuff permanently affixed to your body, stealing your life away, is okay with you, then that's your prerogative, but at least now you'll be going through life with your eyes open. It's one thing to make a choice and live life accordingly, freely accepting the consequences of these choices, it's another thing entirely to live life with your eyes closed.

They, Who?

Recent news reports are declaring that some people have suffered heart attacks as a result of taking Vioxx, a drug that was prescribed to reduce inflammation caused by certain types of arthritis. Like those who went before them with various other diseases or illnesses caused by some product or drug, the afflicted will cry out, "But they said it was safe."

My question to all these people is, "They, who?" The meat and dairy industries? Pharmaceutical companies? The AMA? The FDA? The government? Drugs are big business, very big business. Once flesh became a product for the masses, enormous amounts of money were at stake, and the meat and dairy industries, professional associations such as the AMA, and even greedy governments want as much of it as they can possibly get their hands on. Do you really believe that your well-being will take priority over their profits and power? Do you really think they care that you'll develop heart disease or cancer? Or do you think they care about today's bottom line? Governmental organizations such as the FDA are made up of doctors and researchers whose jobs are to promote and *enforce* the further use of doctors and researchers. They are a self-serving advocacy group, and are not selfless purveyors of truth. Caveat emptor.

But don't blame them for your bad health. Nobody's forcing you to continue to eat a poisonous product now that you know the facts. We must make our health and well-being our individual responsibility, and becoming vegan is the ultimate way of accepting this responsibility. Making the switch to veganism is very empowering, and when you hear people say, "But they said ...," you'll be proud that you no longer need to resort to the all-too-popular abdication of personal responsibility.

Miscellaneous Meat Maladies

Other diseases and conditions that can be a direct result of our meat-based diet are gout, arthritis, eye disorders, allergies, acid-reflux, constipation, multiple sclerosis, Alzheimer's disease, epilepsy and birth defects, to name a few. Even diseases that cannot be directly attributable to a meat-based diet and do not quickly reverse when a vegan regimen is used are undoubtedly precipitated by many of the factors brought about by a meat-eating, meat-producing world. Mad cow disease, avian flu, salmonella and many other calamities are being wrought upon our society because of meat-eating lifestyles.

> *"Nothing will benefit human health and increase the chances for survival of life on Earth as much as the evolution to a vegetarian diet."*   – Albert Einstein

Conventional Health

It is extremely important to keep in mind that health is not so much a "possessable" chemical equation, as it is currently looked upon by conventional medicine. To the greatest extent, health is a state of being that is simply an extension of a lifestyle. Live according to nature and be healthy, or live in contrast to nature and health becomes a much sought after, and heavily researched, concept. Meat eaters can engage in the folly of pursuing health, but cannot ever achieve it.

The laws of nature are clear: Veganism for all mankind.

Chapter 18

The Environment

"You must teach your children that the ground beneath their feet is the ashes of our grandfathers. So that they will respect the land, tell your children that the Earth is rich with the lives of our kin. Teach your children what we have taught our children, that the Earth is our mother. Whatever befalls the Earth befalls the sons of the Earth. If men spit upon the ground, they spit upon themselves. This we know, the Earth does not belong to man – man belongs to the Earth. All things are connected like the blood which unites one family. Whatever befalls the Earth befalls the sons of the Earth. Man did not weave the web of life, he is merely a strand in it. Whatever he does to the web, he does to himself."
– The character of Chief Seattle,
as written by Ted Perry in the movie *Home*

What is truly good for one person is good for all people. What is truly good for all people is good for one person. Nowhere is this more evident than when we consider the Earth's environment – our home of homes.

To many people, environmental matters can seem abstract and distant from anything whatsoever to do with them. After all, the rain forests are so far away, who cares if they're cut down and burned? "No skin off my nose." Sadly, there are many entities that rely on this apathy for their continued power and money. But the truth is, maintaining a healthy environment is critical to your own health and happiness. Everyone should have an understanding of our environment, its ecosystems and the importance of maintaining them. The more you know, the more you will help yourself. The more you help yourself, the more you help the Earth and all who reside here.

Everyone Is Downstream From Someone

If you've ever had an aquarium containing tropical fish you may know that aquariums are their own ecosystem of recycling and rejuvenation. Fish eat and produce waste, which is deposited on the gravel at the bottom of the tank. The under-gravel filter slowly draws this waste through the gravel and breaks it down into small particles. Bacteria (good bacteria) present within this ecosystem assist in the decomposition. Once the broken-down waste is small enough to be drawn into the filter, it has already begun changing from waste into basic chemical elements. As these elements pass through the filter, the waste becomes completely neutralized. What was once waste material has now become a usable and valuable source of food for the plants and, in turn, the fish in the aquarium. It is a cyclical system with no end and no beginning.

Our planet has many ecosystems, and all of these small ecosystems comprise our environment. Each aspect of the environment – air, land, water, vegetation, etc. – plays a role in the continual cycle. When one link breaks, so goes the chain, and so goes life as we know it. Fortunately (or maybe unfortunately), it doesn't happen in a day. We are paying for our parents' misguided ways and our children will pay for ours, until such time as we go bankrupt – and this kind of bankruptcy can't be discharged with all the money in the world.

> *"Most people are largely unaware of the wide-ranging effects cattle are having on the ecosystems of the planet and the fortunes of civilization. Yet, cattle production and beef consumption now rank among the gravest threats to the future well-being of the Earth and its human population."*
> – Jeremy Rifkin

The consumption of meat by the human race is breaking many links in our ecosystems. If the current trends in levels of meat production and consumption continue, then an environmental, cataclysmic end of life as we know it could come within the next fifty to one hundred years. And while this can seem like an overly exaggerated claim, the fact is, the planet can simply not sustain this rate of destruction. In a ferocious attempt at justifying The Big Lie, many meat eaters resort to saying things like, "Well, lions eat meat, so why aren't they responsible for any of the damage?" The answer, and truth, is lions and other "natural" carnivores perform a very valuable role within their ecosystem. They are a vacuum cleaner of sorts, cleaning the Earth of what would be dying and rotting flesh. They help keep the ecosystem clean by converting what necessarily dies back into life. For humans to consume flesh means something quite different and, in fact, is the exact opposite of lions. We are utilizing many of the Earth's resources to create life solely in order to kill it. In short, by eating meat, lions take death and turn it into life; humans take life and turn it into death.

We kill over ten billion animals a year, and this killing cycle yields ever-diminishing returns from the resources of the Earth. The results are alterations or, more accurately, aberrations in the cycles of the environment. These aberrations invade every fiber of the Earth's existence and, consequently, our existence. Disease, pollution, etc., none of which are necessarily inherent in life, are mutational products of this unnatural lifestyle.

To Compost Or Not To Compost (Meat Is The Difference)

A backyard compost is a heap of vegetable matter and discards, such as grass clippings, cabbage leaves, coffee grounds or an old carrot you found in the back of the refrigerator. This vegetable matter decomposes into what looks very much like soil. In fact, vegetable matter decomposes into the basic elements that created the vegetable matter in the first place. This compost is rich in nutrients and makes a wonderful fertilizer for your garden. Again, this is another link in an ecosystem – vegetable matter that becomes food for more vegetables.

Meat and animal products cannot be put into a typical compost heap because meat does not break down in the same way vegetable matter does. Meat is putrefactive. It literally rots as it decays, creating bad bacteria. Flesh that is left out on soil to decompose can actually be injurious to the soil. If you had a nice green lawn and threw a steak on it, the grass surrounding the steak may turn yellow and die. On the other hand, if you threw an apple core on the lawn, it would decompose into matter the lawn would use as fertilizer (and you may even end up with a new apple tree, which produces still more food).

> *"What can I compost? Most yard waste, like grass clippings, fallen leaves, twigs, vines and plant stalks, can be composted. Fruits and vegetable scraps, coffee grounds and nutshells can also be composted ... You should never compost meat, fish, poultry, dairy products."* – GreenTreks.org

Let's consider cow manure for a moment. Okay, a brief moment. Cow manure is valuable fertilizer because the cow is a herbivore. If you fed meat to a cow, the excrement would no longer be usable as fertilizer. Conversely, human feces (from a meat eater) is putrefactive and toxic, inhibiting and destroying our ecosystems still further. By becoming vegan, you support the Earth's natural ecosystems, even by eating. As a vegan, your waste is no longer destructive to the environment, nor are you contributing to ever-diminishing returns. Your excrement is now valuable fertilizer, as opposed to putrefactive waste and disease-producing sewage. No matter how much you eat, you aren't detracting from the Earth's finite resources. You are just a link in the never-ending cycle of life.

Diminishing Returns

Eating meat and animal products is a prime example of the law of diminishing returns. It takes roughly twelve pounds of grain (as cattle feed) to produce one pound of hamburger. Twelve pounds of grain as bread or cereal can feed a heck of a lot more people than one pound of meat. On top of this, we must consider the cycle of life and the ecosystems our food choices affect. Eat a vegan regimen, and the life cycle continues. Eat meat, and the life cycle continues to break down.

Vegans grow twelve pounds of grain to eat twelve pounds of grain, which produces twelve pounds of waste, which becomes fertilizer for another twelve pounds of grain. Meat eaters grow twelve pounds of grain to produce one pound of meat. They eat this one pound of meat and produce one pound of putrefactive and environmentally hazardous waste, which inhibits growing more grain.

It takes a considerable amount of land to produce twelve pounds of grain. Imagine, then, how much land you need in order to produce enough food for the world at a ratio of twelve pounds of grain to one pound of meat. Another way to look at this is that one acre of land will yield 165 pounds of beef – or 20,000 pounds of potatoes. The meat eaters have to continually find more land that hasn't been destroyed by meat and its waste. We are running out of land that can sustain life because of meat.

Our planet is currently experiencing worldwide wheat shortages, in part because of this 12:1 grain to meat ratio (and for other reasons you are about to learn). World hunger is a direct result of meat consumption. Eating meat and animal products supports the use of vegetable matter to produce meat which, in turn, inhibits the further production of vegetable matter, ever diminishing returns to the point where food becomes scarce and, eventually, nonexistent. On the other hand, producing food for vegans automatically requires twelve times less land, plus the land continues to sustain plant growth. Being vegan means a never-ending supply of vegetation for a never-ending supply of food for a never-ending supply of vegetation for a never-ending supply of food ...

McDonald's And The Rain Forests

Unfortunately, little in this world is held sacred anymore. Just about any marketing or advertising executive will tell you that anything goes in order to sell a product. Perhaps one of the most unscrupulous of all atrocities is served up by McDonald's.

The rain forests are so far away and seem to have no bearing on our comfortable lives. But it just so happens that the rain forests produce much of the world's oxygen, filter our waters and are home to many species of plants and animals that are vital to our ecosystems in some ways of which we aren't even yet aware. Fortunately, more and more people are becoming aware of the enormous value and necessity of the rain forests. It has even become fashionable to wear "Save The Rain Forests" T-shirts, so fashionable that even McDonald's decided to get in on the act, promoting rain forest awareness with a range of toys that came with their meals. So what's the big McDeal? The deal is, saying "Save the rain forests" does nothing to save the rain forests.

Official estimates vary, but it is safe to say that roughly ninety percent of all rain forest destruction is to clear land to grow feed for livestock. Let me repeat that. Rain forests are being destroyed to produce meat. Eating meat equals destruction of the rain forests. Consider that there were once four billion acres of rain forest, and we are now destroying an area twice the size of Florida every year. Already fifty percent is gone forever. At this current rate, there will be no more rain forests by the year 2060. And even if you don't care about the biodiversity, potential life-saving herbs and indigenous people's habitat, you might care to remember that without trees you will have no oxygen to breathe. What happens when our rain forests are gone? Where will we get our oxygen? Oxygen-R-Us, perhaps? Perhaps not.

McDonald's selling rain forest toys is akin to Jeffrey Dahmer carving figurines of his victims and then offering them to their families as reminders of their beloved. It is a deranged practice, and perhaps even another intentional smoke screen.

I'm glad everyone is talking about saving the rain forests. I hope more and more people learn what is really responsible for the forests' demise. But talking about saving the rain forests over a Big Mac or Whopper is an absurd contrariety. The best way to save the rain forests, in fact the only way to save the rain forests, is to eliminate animals from the menu. It's also the only way to save yourself, your family and all future generations.

The Solution To World Hunger Is Only A Burger Away

People are starving because humans eat meat. The same twelve pounds of grain it takes to produce one pound of hamburger can make twenty-four plates of spaghetti. Cattle consume seventy percent of all the grain produced in this country. Sending a donation to a world hunger charity while eating a steak is one of life's funny little wastes of time. Save your money and eat spaghetti (or any plant food) instead. This will save the hungry from dying. If you don't follow this simple plan, the group of hungry will eventually include you or your children. No matter how much money you may accumulate, there will simply be no food to buy. Like it or not, it is no more complex than that. Even if you could find a tomato, the ground will have been depleted of its ability to grow more tomatoes.

If you truly care about the hungry and want to see world hunger curtailed, you need to do something that will create a more abundant food supply. You need to give up meat and animal products. That's just the way it is.

Not A Drop To Drink

Drinkable water, once in abundant supply, is becoming a scarce commodity. Little wonder, when you consider how much water it takes to produce meat and animal products. John Robbins, in his book *May All Be Fed*, put together the following chart:

Water needed to produce one pound of:	
Tomatoes	23 Gallons
Lettuce	23 Gallons
Potatoes	24 Gallons
Wheat	25 Gallons
Carrots	33 Gallons
Apples	49 Gallons
Eggs	544 Gallons
Chicken	815 Gallons
Pork	1,630 Gallons
Beef	5,214 Gallons

Fully half of all the water consumed in the United States is used to provide drinking water and to grow feed for cattle and other livestock. Of the water that's left, virtually all of it is contaminated, thanks to our meat-eating ways.

Americans produce about twelve thousand pounds of excrement every second, excrement that, as we've learned, is putrefactive and destructive to the environment. Our once pristine, drinkable waters are now little more than a large, toxic, putrefactive sewer system. Moreover, when one pound of beef or chicken or any animal product is consumed, the waste becomes harmful to the groundwater and, therefore, the environment, and inhibits further food production. When one pound of plant food is consumed, the waste becomes fertilizer for more plant food.

Just twenty years ago I had never yet sipped bottled water. Now, like many people, I have serious concerns about even brushing my teeth with tap water. Shouldn't this be telling us something alarming? The good news is we don't need to pass more laws or have heftier governmental budgets. We just need to take responsibility for our own actions.

A few years ago there was a television commercial for a drinking water company whose slogan was intriguing. While you were looking at a delicious waterfall in an idyllic mountain setting, the voiceover said, "If we all lived here, we could all have water this fresh." The message was, since we don't live "here" we need to buy their product. What is sadly fascinating is that if we all did, in fact, live "here," that fresh water they speak of would be polluted by our lifestyle. The filthy water where we now live wasn't filthy before we all moved here.

The Recycling Game

It has become quite fashionable to recycle. Cans, bottles, newspapers and the like are being recycled by the ton. This is a positive step, but let's put things into their proper perspective. The well-meaning person who recycles yet eats meat is a lot like someone who drinks diet cola to wash down a cheeseburger and ice cream sundae. One cannot truly be an environmentalist while eating animals and animal products.

Recycling is a wonderful technology, but it does practically nothing to save an otherwise doomed environment. Saran Wrap is not our real problem, folks. What does, in fact, doom our environment is what the Saran Wrap is wrapping – animal parts. Meat production and consumption is literally decimating our planet. Whereas recycling may move us one step forward, eating animals takes the environment *many* steps back.

In a vegan world, recycling becomes a valuable aid to our ecosystems, as ecosystems themselves are a process of recycling. But because meat production and consumption are diminishing the planet's life-sustaining resources, recycling while continuing to produce and consume meat is nothing but sheer folly. Eating meat is causing the breakdown of the Earth's ecosystems, worldwide deforestation, topsoil erosion and numerous other calamities. No matter how many bottles are recycled, the world will still not be able to maintain life without forests, topsoil, pure water and oxygen. Giving up animal products is the only thing you can do that will actually save the environment.

Become vegan and recycling is an environmental benefit. Continue eating meat and all the recycling in the world won't amount to a pile of beans. (No pun intended. Well, maybe.)

Arbor Day It Ain't

"The road to hell is paved with good intention."
                                    – Late 16th Century proverb

Charitable organizations are an interesting phenomenon. More than they actually help society, charities help society to *believe* something positive is being done. In reality, charities are similar to any going concern, in that they need to maintain a cash flow. They, too, pay salaries, rent, insurance, utilities, etc. Instead of selling a product to gain this revenue, charities simply sell a cause.

While there are countless charitable workers seeking a better world, the results they're looking for can only be realized by aligning themselves with, and promoting, truth, nature and, therefore, veganism. Heart disease would be virtually nonexistent in a vegan world. So why doesn't the American Heart Association promote veganism and do all it can to expose the dangers of a meat-eating lifestyle? Many cancers would be eliminated in a vegan world. So why doesn't the American Cancer Society promote veganism? Type 2 diabetes affects millions of people, holding them captive to a life of drugs and/or injections. This form of diabetes can be reversed with a change to a vegan diet. So why doesn't the American Diabetes Association do anything to promote this awareness? The answer is as simple as it is difficult to swallow.

Several years ago, I saw a commercial for the National Arbor Day Foundation (NADF), which speaks out against deforestation and asks for contributions so they can plant trees. What are contributions going to do while the masses still eat meat? Never once during their commercial did they say stop eating meat and animal products, yet this is the chief culprit of deforestation. I have a nagging hunch that most, if not all, of the folks at the NADF eat meat.

> *"Amount of U.S. land that could be returned to forest for each American who adopts a meat-free diet: 35,000 square feet."*   – *May All Be Fed*, by John Robbins

Thirty-five thousand square feet of U.S. land are at stake for each and every American, and this doesn't even take into consideration the tropical rain forests, which are being cut down and burned at a frenzied pace. In the United States alone, not to mention the rain forests, almost two hundred million acres of land could be returned to forest if Americans gave up eating animals and animal products. For every one step the NADF hopes to move us forward, meat eating moves us exponentially backwards. The NADF can put on a TV commercial showing a cluster of people planting a handful of trees and it appears so nice and beneficial, while meat eating is decimating our planet's forests.

While the road to hell is, in fact, paved with good *intention*, life rewards *action*. Veganism is the asphalt on the road to paradise. Giving up meat and animal products and turning to a plant-based diet is the only way for our planet to win, which helps us to win, which helps the planet to win, which helps us to win …

Pesticides Are Suicide

Humans manufacture pesticides predominantly because we need to grow vast amounts of grain to fatten livestock. The idea is that less of the crop is lost to insects. This is a Pandora's Box of calamities.

For one thing, the pesticide doesn't stay on the crops. Most of it gets into the soil, then into the groundwater and then into our drinking water supplies and oceans, from which all the Earth's inhabitants drink. In most cases, drinking water means ingesting pesticides. Then, to add further insult to injury, consuming animals means consuming concentrated pesticides that the animals have accumulated in their flesh over the course of their lives from the pesticide-treated grain they've eaten.

Pesticides are biocidal, which means they kill life. We are life. We get killed. It may not be instantaneous; we don't fall to the floor flailing our limbs in a desperate attempt for our last breath. It's more insidious than that. Eat a hamburger and, in addition to fat, blood, urine, hormones, antibiotics and a host of other goodies, you're consuming even more concentrated pesticides. Is it any wonder why birth defects are soaring? I wonder why organizations such as the March Of Dimes don't encourage people to stop eating animals. Instead of generating huge amounts of revenue (and ensuring this revenue forever), promoting veganism would actually curtail and possibly eliminate birth defects.

The "experts" don't understand why degenerative disease and birth defects are proliferating simply because they eat animal products and are lifetime subscribers to The Big Lie. The answers are sitting on their dinner plates, and they're looking everywhere else.

The truth is about eighty percent of all pesticides is used on crops to be used as feed for livestock. And we're talking about billions of tons of pesticides. By everyone becoming vegan, eighty percent of pesticides will *automatically* be eliminated. Then, because so much less land is needed to produce crops, we won't need to be so concerned about getting every bit out of each acre. This would allow for more organic produce, that is, produce that is grown entirely without pesticides.

More and more marine animals are dying from "unknown" causes. "Red tide" kills zillions of marine animals and, again, nobody knows why. If you have never seen an outbreak of red tide, I can tell you from first-hand experience that the beaches are blanketed with dead fish. Even people get sick from red tide, just by walking by the beach. Our coral reefs are vanishing and our experts are stumped.

Is it really that hard to understand? It's actually easy to understand from the proper perspective. The truth is, pesticides, putrefactive waste from meat eaters, topsoil erosion and the like are invading our waters and oceans and destroying the water's ability to sustain life. All of these environmental catastrophes have their basis almost exclusively in animal product production and consumption. To top it all off, many insects and bad bacteria proliferate in the rotting, putrefactive environment created by animal products. A meat-eating world believes it needs to manufacture more and more pesticides, but it is the very lifestyle that is causing much of the problem. By becoming vegan, insect control becomes nearly automatic.

I would bet anyone a trillion apples that if the world went vegan, red tide would diminish, coral reefs would come back to life, heart disease, diabetes, cancer and birth defects would immediately decline and eventually vanish. So would a lot of nonprofit organizations.

Topsoil: A Top Priority

It takes nature and her ecosystems hundreds of years to produce one inch of topsoil. As a result of meat and animal products we are now losing one inch of topsoil every sixteen years. If the human race continues producing and consuming animal products, it won't be long before there is no usable land to grow food.

The United Sates is a strong nation because of, in part, our vast natural resources. Our croplands once had more than twenty inches of topsoil. They now have about six or seven inches. It's just a matter of time before there is none.

> *"An inch of topsoil takes between 200 and 1,000 years to form under natural conditions. With the human and cattle population growing at an unprecedented rate, it seems that virtually every available square mile of rangeland and cropland is being exploited, depleted, and eroded with little thought of tomorrow or the needs of future generations." – Beyond Beef*, by Jeremy Rifkin

Worldwide deforestation is underway to enable us to produce meat. Deforestation facilitates increasing topsoil erosion. Therefore, topsoil loss is directly attributable to meat production. As forests vanish, leaving nothing to stabilize the topsoil, the topsoil erodes into our water supply and oceans.

Topsoil belongs not in water, but on land. When topsoil enters the water supply it fouls the water and greatly decreases the ocean's ability to sustain life. Increasingly, the planet is experiencing desertification, ever-increasing deserts and dust bowls that cannot grow crops. Desertification is directly attributable to meat production.

The Byzantine world of biotechnology is now stepping in to offer "solutions" to a planet that is facing worldwide food shortages. You should, by now, know that this is really just problematic and inept problem solving and will only serve to confuse the issue, while the world implodes. The relationships between biotechnology and meat are interestingly interwoven. In a vegan world, biotechnology would be seen for the evil folly it is. In a meat-eating world, biotechnology steps in to offer new ways to supply food, since meat eating is destroying the old ways. Again, let the buyer beware.

We must hope that the window of opportunity has not yet closed and proceed as if it may close tomorrow. If mankind gives up meat and turns to a vegan diet, not only would the diminishing returns effect of meat be stopped but natural composting would eventually replenish our topsoil supply. In turn, food availability would stabilize and even rise, supplying food for all the Earth's inhabitants. Moreover, the waters would also return to their drinkable, life-sustaining condition.

Global Warming

Millions of years ago there were organisms that absorbed carbons out of the air. This actually paved the way for man, who obviously needed an abundance of oxygen rather than carbon. As these creatures died and their remains returned to the ground, these carbons were contained deep inside the Earth. The burning of fossil fuels – natural gas, oil and coal – releases these carbons back into the atmosphere.

Before man began burning fossil fuel, the Sun's rays would penetrate the Earth's outer atmosphere and then bounce off the Earth, back into space. Now, however, this carbon has created something of a cloud so that when the Sun's powerful rays enter the atmosphere they are no longer able to exit. They are trapped by what is called the "greenhouse effect." This results in global warming. One-third of the United States' natural resources are utilized in the production of animal products. By abstaining from using animal products you help to drastically reduce the amount of carbon being disbursed into the atmosphere.

The burning of the rain forests is also a chief culprit in dispensing carbon back into the atmosphere. Moreover, each tree that is cut down is one less tree that can convert carbon dioxide into oxygen for us to breathe.

Pro Life

There are many well-intentioned people who consider themselves to be environmentalists, and yet many of these people eat animal products, even though it is animal products that are primarily responsible for the demise of the environment. Eating meat kills animals, people and the planet. To be an environmentalist, one must be vegan. We should all be true environmentalists because the planet is our home of homes.

Isn't it time to stop the killing? Isn't it time to choose life for ourselves, our neighbors and our planet? Turning to a vegan diet is the essence of life for the environment and all who reside herein.

Veganism is to life for our planet, whereas meatism is to its death. Which will you choose? Which will you work toward?

Chapter 19

Jobs

It seems that almost every discussion about matters of the environment brings up the issue of jobs. For instance, every argument about the environmental ramifications of deforestation in the United States is met with a counter-argument, not on the environmental impact, but on the loss of jobs for people engaged in cutting down the trees. There are many jobs that function, directly or otherwise, in an environmentally destructive fashion. Cutting down trees, commercial fishing, slaughtering animals and the like employ many people, and to concern oneself altruistically with the environment can seem to be insensitive to people's livelihoods. This, in itself, can offer insight into why problems are proliferating – true problem solving is politically incorrect.

Sometimes it can appear as though being altruistic on one side of the equation is being callous on the other side. This is a dangerous belief that fosters further growth of The Big Lie. Is it callousness if a society embraces freedom, frowns upon control of freedom and then fights against a control-hungry regime? This fight can (and will) be labeled callousness by the control-hungry regime looking to foist their own subjective ways upon the world. This fight, however, is not an offensive sword, but rather a shield to protect what is a divine and unalienable right to all who reside on the planet.

"The shepherd drives the wolf from the sheep's throat, for which the sheep thanks the shepherd as his liberator, while the wolf denounces him for the same act, as the destroyer of liberty, especially since the sheep was a black one. Plainly, the sheep and the wolf are not agreed upon a definition of the word liberty; and precisely the same difference prevails today among us human creatures."
— Abraham Lincoln

From Tree Chopper To Tree Hugger

In the pursuit of what is just and good, any and all jobs that are destroying the environment should be expunged. What true value is there in a job that is harmful to the planet? A job must be productive not only for the employed, but for those affected by the employment. As we now know, what is truly good for one is good for all, and what is truly good for all is good for one. Violating this basic tenet of life will pejoratively transcend all aspects of life on the planet, whereas living in accordance with this tenet will yield life, health, humanity and prosperity, as nature intended.

People who have jobs that are counterproductive to a healthy and sane planet won't be out of work for long, because there are a great many other jobs that can be created to restore our planet to health. People who once cut down trees, for example, could become stewards of the land, planting and caring for new forests. In fact, they would be the best suited.

"Our wholeness as human beings depends upon the depth of our awareness of the fact that we are a part of the wholeness of nature."
— Ashley Montagu

Those engaged in, or in support of, deforestation claim that "tree huggers" simply have nothing better to do, so they care more about the trees than they do people's livelihoods. In actuality, what is far more probable is that the tree choppers have kept so busy that they haven't had any time to consider the truth and the ramifications of their work. The pursuit of money can keep us all far too busy to think and, therefore, too busy to care about the truly important things; certainly far too busy to consider why society is structured this way in the first place. There are many entities that like keeping people too busy to think. Then, those who are kept too busy to think resent those who take the time to think. This resentment polarizes people and moves society that much farther from the truth. Resentment, anger and debate proliferate, while health and humanity lie in ruins.

Help Wanted: Doomsday Director

"We are seeking a candidate to fill the position of World Doomsday Director. The successful candidate will be responsible for finding and implementing a method of destroying the world."

If there was such an opening, I suspect the world would be outraged. I would hope that society would not only not sanction such a job but do everything possible to eliminate it. I'm happy to report there is no such job with that specific title or job description (that I know about), but I am very sorry to report there are many actual jobs bringing about the same effect.

Why are we not outraged? Why are we not doing everything in our power to correct the misguided?

Brute Force Doesn't Tread Lightly

A meat-eating society needs people to fill jobs such as slaughterer (to provide meat), tree-chopper (to clear land to grow feed for this meat), medical researchers experimenting on innocent animals (to supposedly find cures for diseases brought about by eating this meat), and doctors (to keep us all primed to continue the cycle). This is part of the job cycle within The Big Lie, and it is an existence made almost entirely of brute force; hardly the essence of treading lightly upon the Earth.

Treading lightly upon the Earth, another key aspect of veganism, is living life as an expression of respect and love for ourselves, each other, our home and our Creator. Treating the Earth as though it is a precious and fragile gift from God is the forbidden finesse the meat-eating world scoffs at so easily while ravaging the planet. But it can only be jobs that reflect this finesse that can create and maintain a happy and healthy planet.

Work For What You Want

How about replacing the old destructive jobs with new jobs that are constructive and beneficial to society? How about jobs that build houses and shelters for all the planet's creatures, not just those with money – or two legs? How about health care jobs that care for, not exploit, all the Earth's inhabitants, such as jobs that would give care and treatment to, say, a deer that gets hit by a car? In this case, those with true health care jobs would care for the deer rather than letting it suffer and die while offering an explanation in financial and sociopathic terms that "it's only a deer." If there were such health care professionals, health care would be provided not only to all deer but to all people. This is far and away from our health care system today. Tom Cruise need not worry, he's in good hands. Tom Smith, however, should be quite concerned.

How about jobs that grow food for all? How about jobs that create new wildlife habitats? How about jobs that bring joy to people of the world in art and entertainment? How about building new methods of environmentally friendly transportation? How about building new roads that are raised above the ground, so millions of animals and people can migrate underneath without risk of being injured or killed when crossing? In simple terms, how about jobs that care about the world, its inhabitants and its future, rather than solely about money? Pursuing something as unnatural as money will never yield what we all think we are working toward – happiness. Having jobs that are subjective and destructive creates a world that reflects subjectivity and destruction. Having jobs that are loving and productive would reflect love and productivity. Which one is better? Actually, "better" is a subjective word, so let me rephrase that. Which one is good?

Becoming, say, a doctor or health care provider out of a desire to care for others, then refusing treatment to those without financial means is a farce. Moreover, jobs that outright destroy the Earth's resources, or jobs that entail murdering billions of animals, are nothing short of evil. Sanctioning and engaging in jobs that kill billions and ravage the planet cannot possibly bring about the kind of world we all claim we want. The horror stories that fill our newspapers are easily understandable from this perspective. Why do we condone and support these jobs?

It has been said that to save one life is to save the world. By being vegan (and having a job aligned with the principles of veganism) one saves many lives: the lives of the animals that are no longer eaten, the lives of the animals that live in forests that are no longer destroyed, the lives of the animals that are no longer brutalized in research laboratories, the lives of the people whose exposure to a meat-eating world has been lessened, the life of the environment, and the life of thyself.

> *"To know even one life has breathed easier because you have lived – this is to have succeeded."*
> – Ralph Waldo Emerson

Mr. Emerson's sentiment is tremendously inspirational, perhaps even more so when one realizes the flip side is also true: To know many lives have suffered because you have lived – this is to have failed.

Getting Ahead Or Losing Ground With Each Step

Many people think they work hard so that they can make money to be able to buy things they want. In many cases, they are overlooking the fact that what they really want is to be happy. They simply believe that what they buy will bring them happiness. Unfortunately, you cannot spend your life fundamentally opposed to the principles of happiness and then go out and buy it. It just doesn't work that way. If you want to be happy, then you need to spend your life aligned with the fundamental and technical aspects of happiness. Pursuing the "American dream" at the expense of humanity will, in the end, only yield nightmares. In a world where many people are trying to get ahead, it is important to remember one thing: One cannot get ahead of happiness. Happiness and humanity are connected – intrinsically so.

Love, peace and harmony for all are universally spoken as ultimate human values, while many jobs are diametrically opposed to realizing these values. Ask yourself if the job you have, your life's work, bespeaks the values you consider important in your life. If you want your life to be productive, loving, caring, happy and spiritually fulfilling in accordance with your God, your life's work needs to reflect that. We're all in your hands. And vice versa.

Mission Possible

Your job, if you choose to accept it, is to know that if you want to live in a paradise, you need to work toward it. Everything you do, and even all the things you don't do, either bring paradise closer or move it farther away. And it all starts with what you put into your mouth.

Part Three

Choose your life:

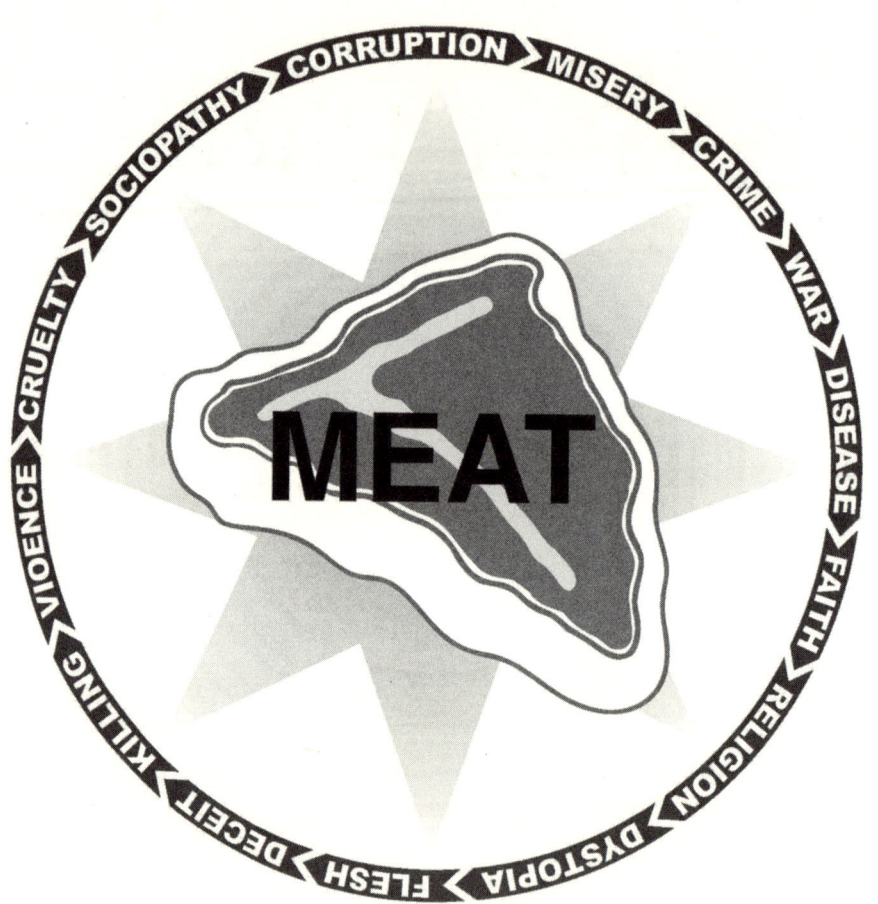

CORRUPTION MISERY CRIME WAR DISEASE FAITH RELIGION DYSTOPIA FLESH DECEIT KILLING VIOENCE CRUELTY SOCIOPATHY

MEAT

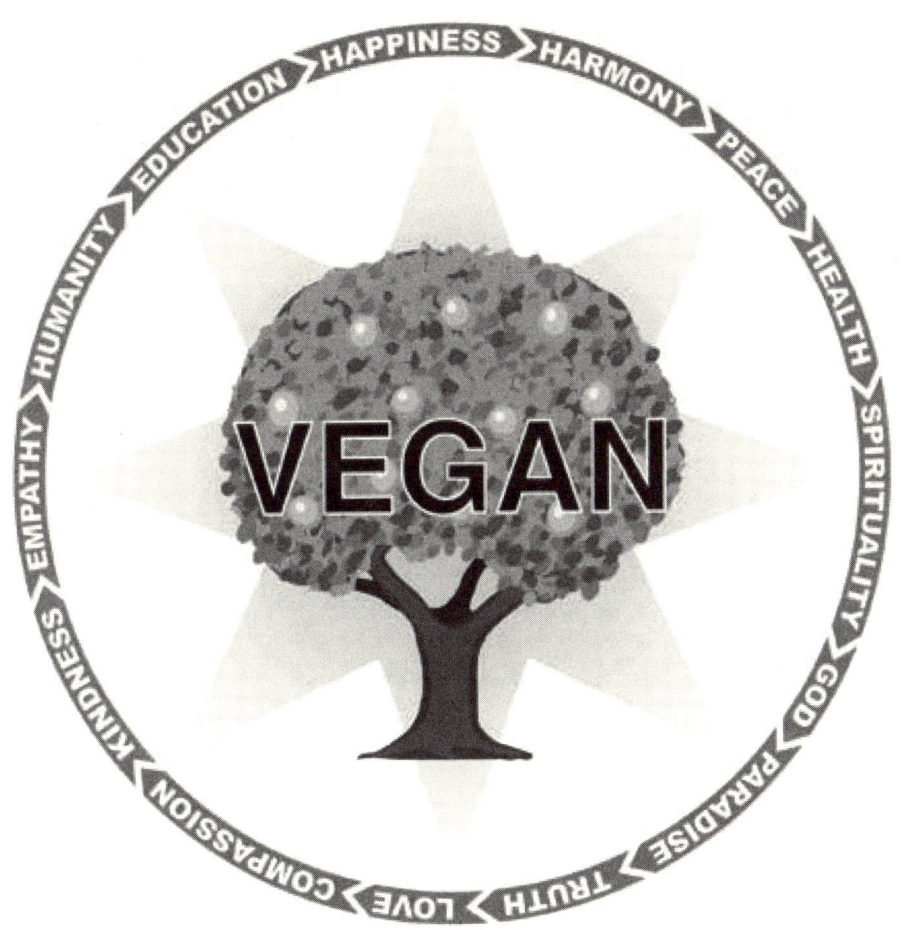

Chapter 20

The Vegan Way

Y ou should now have a clear understanding of why it is critically important that you (and every man, woman and child on the planet) be vegan. But we're not quite done. It is also important to understand how to implement that knowledge. Whereas the book, up to this point, has been all about the "whys," *The Vegan Way* is all about the "hows." This chapter will discuss products to use and products to avoid – some of which you may find quite surprising. Further, and more importantly, it will offer additional suggestions and resources for a lifelong journey of learning. Be aware that even if you are determined to be vegan immediately, it can still take some time to rid your life of animal products. It is a process of learning and enlightenment.

Right Now

The very first thing you should do is to promise yourself you will never again swallow the flesh of an animal – any animal. The good news is that today there are plenty of delicious options available for anyone becoming vegan. It's no longer just tofu or lentils for the rest of your life. In fact, you can still eat just about all the same meals you eat today by substituting any animal product ingredients with meat-free and dairy-free alternatives. That means vegan alternatives to bacon, sausage, hamburgers, hot dogs, pizzas, fish, beef, chicken, turkey, milk, cheese, ice cream and anything else that you currently enjoy are still on the menu, with many of the ingredients, and even fully-prepared meals, widely available in your local supermarket and/or health food store. Take a look in the refrigerated section and you will also find vegan substitutes for sandwich meats such as ham, bologna, turkey, chicken, salami, pastrami, etc. Also, don't forget that much of the food you eat now is already vegan, such as cereal, pasta, rice, potatoes and all fruit and vegetables, so it will not be as difficult or intimidating as it may appear initially.

Go get some vegan cookbooks and find some recipes you'll enjoy preparing and eating. As a rule of thumb, if a cookbook has one recipe that you'll incorporate into your repertoire of weekly meals, that is a worthwhile book. If you don't want to spend money on buying lots of books, you can try your local library or, if you have Internet access, go online and search for "vegan recipes." You'll find a cornucopia of resources on new and exciting meal suggestions.

You must stock your house right away with foods that will satisfy you, or you will reach for the familiar animal products of the past. In addition to the obvious fruits, vegetables, grains, nuts and legumes, you may wish to try some of the increasingly available meat substitutes, as many of these are indistinguishable from the "real thing" and may ease your transition to a natural and humane lifestyle. As with any food, though, there will be some that you like and some that you don't, so don't reject all veggie burgers just because you try one that doesn't suit you. Experiment, and you'll find there are many products out there you absolutely love.

Avoid, Avoid, Avoid:

Eat no flesh, no milk, no cheese, no yogurt, no eggs. Also, eat nothing containing gelatin (from animal bone), whey or casein (milk byproducts) or "natural flavors" (usually means chicken broth). Read the ingredients on everything you buy and avoid anything with ingredients you don't fully recognize, as many foods that appear to be vegan may contain animal products.

Every time you drive past a McDonalds, Burger King, Wendy's, etc., and are tempted to stop in "just this once," allow truth to replace denial and remind yourself of what these places really are – morgues.

You should also avoid any form of exploitation of animals, such as rodeos, horse or dog races, zoos, aquariums and circuses that include animal acts.

No Skin Off My Nose

What would you say of me if I said we should kill your friends and make lampshades from their skin? So then, what should I say of you who kills my friends and makes lampshades from their skin?

All but the most cold-blooded and sociopathic shun fur coats these days, but even many of these people wear silk, wool and leather. Clothing, bedding and even the upholstery in automobiles comes from sociopathic murder. You should work toward the complete elimination of all animal products from your life.

The meat industries have found a way to profit from something on which they would have otherwise needed to spend billions of dollars dumping into landfills. Clever (and deceptive) marketing has created a belief that leather is a luxury item, and the meat industries are laughing all the way to the bank. (The rest of us should be crying.) Leather is a product of violence and, therefore, should be expunged immediately from society. People love to talk about how leather "breathes." Leather is skin, and skin breathes when it's alive, not dead.

There are many nonleather materials that are far superior to leather that can be used to make shoes, car seats or any other application you can think of. But leather, or more appropriately animal skin, is very cheap at the wholesale level (because so many people are eating the animals' flesh), so manufacturers of shoes and upholstery make more money from leather than they do other materials. Gullible consumers insist on this "luxury" item of death and the manufacturers are only too happy to oblige. Most people in our society claim to love animals, yet are usually making that claim while wearing or sitting on murdered skin. It is abhorrent.

Leather is not a luxury item, it is a product of violence and murder. You should buy shoes made from canvas or any other plant-based or man-made material. The same goes for belts, wallets, handbags, etc. Similarly, you should not buy cars with interiors that use the skin of murdered animals. The principles of love and of God should be more alluring and important than the allure of that shiny Mercedes with the leather interior. If they are not, then you can't ever be upset if someone does something to you that you don't think is "right." They're simply behaving the same way you are. You become their target, as the animal whose skin you want has become your target.

Leather (nor silk, nor wool, etc.) does not exist in paradise.

Cleanliness Is Next To Godliness

The first thing many of us do in the morning is take a shower or a bath. Sadly, however, most people are not getting clean. Imagine if you killed an animal, took its fat, mixed that fat with some perfume and rubbed it all over your body. Would you consider yourself clean? That is essentially how most people "clean" themselves today.

Almost all bar soaps available in supermarkets and drug stores are made from animal fat, although you wouldn't know it from looking at their ingredients. In an effort to not turn people off their products, manufacturers call the animal fat "tallow" or "sodium tallowate," which is essentially animal fat mixed with salt, and it is usually the first ingredient in their soap. Dial, Zest, Irish Spring, SafeGuard and, yes, even "gentle" Dove and the 99 44/100% pure Ivory are all made with animal fat. Though you may have previously thought you were getting clean, you should know that you were simply helping the meat industries clean themselves of all the fat they would have otherwise had to throw away.

Taking a shower and rubbing animal fat on your body only leaves you in need of another shower. Using animal fat to cleanse oneself is vile and further problematic. Even if you eat a vegan diet but still use tallow-based soap, your body is not vegan. Skin is very absorbent, and animal fat rubbed on the skin will enter your body. From a health standpoint, this may very well tend to elevate one's cholesterol levels (animal fat is pretty much nothing but cholesterol). Of course, you shouldn't be surprised that none of the "experts" are saying this, as we now know they are not, in fact, experts.

Have you ever touched poison ivy? If you have, you'll know all too well that the poison doesn't just irritate the skin at the point of contact, but rather it makes your entire body itch. The irritant enters your bloodstream through the skin and circulates through your entire body. I have personal knowledge of people who simply stopped using animal-fat soaps, with no other changes in their diet, and have had a reduction in their serum cholesterol levels. (By the way, if you should ever be afflicted by poison ivy or poison oak, drinking apple juice can completely ease the irritation. Drinking at least several glasses of apple juice each day for the duration of what would be the irritation – sometimes up to two weeks – can completely alleviate the itching.)

Cleanliness is next to Godliness, as the saying goes, and the way to true cleanliness is pretty simple. In addition to not eating animal products, of course, avoid all soaps that list tallow or one of its forms as an ingredient. Also, avoid all bar soaps that don't list all of their ingredients, as it is almost certain that in being evasive the manufacturer has something to hide. Fortunately, it is becoming easier to find bar soaps that use vegetable, plant or fruit oils as their base. This ingredient is usually listed as sodium palmate (palm oil and salt) or something similar, as well as vegetable glycerin (as opposed to glycerin derived from animal fat). You may need to go to health or natural food stores to find these plant-based soaps today but, as demand increases, they will become more widely available.

You cannot rub animal fat on your body and be clean, no matter how nice the factory makes it smell. Why wouldn't everyone make this switch to plant-based soap? If you do, you will be clean, you may get healthier and you may even get closer to God. After all, cleanliness is next to Godliness.

And while we're on the subject, you may or may not be aware that the stunning red lipstick you apply several times a day is also made from, among other things, dead animals. In fact, most mass market cosmetics and household products contain animal products and/or are tested on captive animals, often in the most horrific ways, such as pouring shampoo into the eyes of rabbits to see if it will burn. Read the product labels carefully. If it doesn't state that it does not contain animal ingredients and was not tested on animals, then it almost certainly does and was. There are plenty of products available today that make a point of not testing on animals or using any animal ingredients.

Do Something

In addition to a vegan diet, relaxation and exercise are both vitally important to maintain a properly functioning body. Find some physical activity that you enjoy doing – then do it, regularly.

Relaxation is frequently overlooked in our frenetic world, but stress is a known antagonist to many ailments, and may even be solely responsible for some. There are several excellent methods of relaxation, such as meditation, yoga, biofeedback, imagery or even prayer. Find one you like and incorporate it into your daily life. You will be amazed at how a ten-minute meditation session in the middle of a busy day can pick you up and calm you down.

And, if at all possible, find a doctor and dentist who are vegan, or at least vegetarian, as they will be far better equipped to help you maintain true, long-term health than someone who is trapped in the machinations of The Big Lie.

And, Finally, A Toast:

Pursue love and happiness in your life and make it the very best it can be. Allow all others to do the same. To Life!

Resources

Books To Read:

Diet for a New America: How Your Food Choices Affect Your Health, Happiness and the Future of Life on Earth, by John Robbins

The China Study: The Most Comprehensive Study of Nutrition Ever Conducted and the Startling Implications for Diet, Weight Loss and Long-Term Health, by T. Colin Campbell, Thomas M. Campbell II

Dr. Dean Ornish's Program for Reversing Heart Disease: The Only System Scientifically Proven to Reverse Heart Disease Without Drugs or Surgery, by Dr. Dean Ornish

Vegan Nutrition: Pure and Simple, by Dr. Michael Klaper

Obligate Carnivore, by Jed Gillen

The Bible (At least page one)

Web Sites To Visit:

Here is a small selection of Web sites that, at time of printing, had some useful information or resources. However, Web sites come and go, so always do a search for "vegan" or "animal-friendly" sites.

Because it has been historically difficult to find all the products and information I wanted as a vegan, I started my

239

own Web site, JeffPopick.com, which you may wish to take a look at. There is a whole new world out there for you. Go find it.

Dairy Product Replacements:
www.SilkIsSoy.com
www.Tofutti.com

Sandwich Meat Replacements:
www.Lightlife.com
www.YvesVeggie.com

Meat Replacements:
www.BocaBurger.com
www.MorningstarFarms.com
www.WorthingtonFoods.com

Cosmetics, Personal Care and Household Products:
www.Veganu.com
www.AubreyOrganics.com
www.Ecover.com
www.LeapingBunny.org

Information, Reference Material and Other Resources:
www.GoVeg.com
www.NotMilk.com
www.PCRM.org
www.TheVegetarianChannel.com
www.TheVegetarianSite.com
www.VeganOutreach.org
www.VegetarianStarterKit.com
www.VegSource.com
www.VRG.org

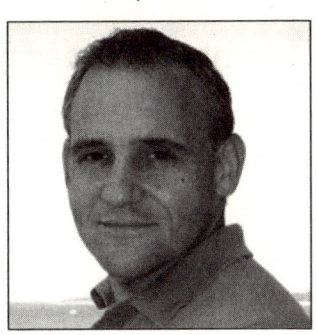

About The Author

Jeff Popick, also known as "The Vegan Sage," is a keen visionary and one of the leading experts on the diverse effects our diet has on our lives and our world. Jeff has worn many hats over the years, from lively radio host to millionaire businessman to passionate author. His latest book, *The Real Forbidden Fruit*, offers a compelling look at how Jeff believes the world was created to be a paradise and the single cause of our demise has been meat. Jeff's assertion is the forbidden fruit was actually meat, and he offers a logical, rational and systematic road map showing the reader how he got there.

Jeff's passion is helping people embrace the principles of veganism and, in so doing, create the paradise the world was originally intended to be. To that end, Jeff is heavily involved in marketing and promoting the vegan message and is also developing healthy and humane vegan products.

Find out more at www.JeffPopick.com.

ORDER FORM

Additional copies of *The Real Forbidden Fruit* in eBook, Hard Cover, Paperback and Audio versions can be ordered from www.TheRealForbiddenFruit.com or by completing the following form and mailing it along with payment to:

VeganWorld Publishing
1083 N. Collier Blvd., #404
Marco Island, FL 34145

· ·

The Real Forbidden Fruit

Paperback ISBN: 978-0-9671518-1-6 $19.95 Qty: _____ Sub total: _____
Hard Cover ISBN: 978-0-9671518-0-9 $29.95 Qty: _____ Sub total: _____
Audio CDs ISBN: 978-0-9671518-2-3 $69.95 Qty: _____ Sub total: _____
Shipping and Handling $4.95 per item Qty: _____ Sub total: _____

TOTAL:_____

Florida residents add 6% sales tax _____ TOTAL: _____

PLEASE PRINT VERY CLEARLY

Name: _____

Street address: _____

City: _____ State: _____ Zip: _____

E-mail address: _____ Phone: _____ Fax: _____

I enclose a check made payable to VeganWorld Publishing for $_____, which includes sales tax, if applicable, and shipping and handling.

OR

Please charge my credit card $_____, which includes sales tax, if applicable, and shipping.

Visa / Mastercard / American Express (circle one)
Card Number:
Expiration Date:
Authorized Signature: _____

Card billing address same as above?   Yes/No
   If "No," please write card billing address here:

_____
_____
_____